a life's
Journey

a life's Journey

Reminiscences, recollections and revelations (1932–2012)

Adrian M Evans

y**L**olfa

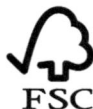

ISBN: 978 184771 641 5

FSC

Published and printed in Wales
on paper from well maintained forests by
Y Lolfa Cyf., Talybont, Ceredigion SY24 5HE
website www.ylolfa.com
e-mail ylolfa@ylolfa.com
tel 01970 832 304
fax 832 782

Acknowledgements

I AM INDEBTED to my family, Edwina, Jill, Trefor and Huw, and to Huw Spencer Lloyd, secretary of Ardwynian Association, for their encouragements, to my brother Trefor Williams Evans, my brother-in-law Brian Macdonald, D Gwyn Williams – my first cousin and Emeritus Professor of Medicine, Guy's, King's and St Thomas's Medical School, King's College, London, my first cousin Gareth Williams and the late Hefin Elias, fellow elder and an Ardwynian, for their sound advice and wise counsel, and especially to Mrs Ann Parry for transforming my handwritten notes for publication.

My story is dedicated to my family.

These reflections were written during 2010 as a therapeutic exercise when I was undergoing chemotherapy treatment for prostate cancer. I recall childhood memories as a son of the manse, and comment on the changing patterns of health care provision in the UK, both as a senior administrator in the NHS and as a consumer of it.

All the proceeds from this publication will be donated to and shared equally with:

Cancer Research Wales, Velindre Hospital, Cardiff, CF14 2TL (Reg Charity No. 248767)

George Thomas Hospice Care, Tŷ George Thomas, Whitchurch Hospital Grounds, Park Road, Whitchurch, Cardiff, CF14 7BF (Reg Charity No. 1023311).

Undesignated gifts will be shared equally with these charities.

Adrian M Evans
March 2013

5

Contents

Forewords

ADRIAN'S MEMOIRS REFLECT aspects of his early life in mid Wales and traces the changing face of healthcare before and since the National Health Service came into being in 1948.

Like all life's journeys, Adrian's had his ups and downs with periods of sadness but mainly very happy times. It is not surprising that in his working life of over 30 years in the NHS he was committed to ensuring that the newly-formed NHS would meet the aspirations of the founders and that, later in life, the NHS proved capable of resolving his own health problems. As a very senior NHS manager, mostly within Wales, he was instrumental in introducing many new procedures to improve patient care. In later years, as a major consumer of the NHS, he highlights some of the challenges facing it.

Cancer Research Wales are very grateful to Adrian and his family for giving half of the proceeds of this book to fund further cancer research in Wales. This book shows how an unselfish commitment to your work, coupled with a strong Christian faith and a very happy family life bring their own reward.

Professor John Moore
President of Cancer Research Wales,
Velindre Cancer Centre

How DIFFICULT IT must be to set out so interesting and fulfilling a life in just a comparatively few pages. There is no doubt that many more interesting events and stories could find their way into his reflections, but what is presented is a story of Adrian's commitment, determination, strength and, dare I say, passion – a passion for public service in the NHS, and what that stands for, the determination to be a meaningful part of that, and the strength to lead others on that sometimes difficult journey. All that is then balanced with the importance of being part of a family, and of living life in line with one's beliefs.

Most such journeys will, from time to time, go through difficult periods. Adrian's honesty in describing his own health problems, and how he has dealt with them, will bring solace and comfort to any who find themselves in a similar position. What comes across is a life of compassion, and a life of caring – caring about family, about friends, and about the countless unknown people who have benefited from Adrian's contribution, over many years, to shaping the NHS we know today. Having spent more than 30 years working in the NHS in Wales myself, I know how valuable that contribution has been.

George Thomas Hospice Care is extremely grateful to Adrian and his family for giving half of the proceeds of this book for the benefit of our patients.

Stephen Harries
Vice-Chairman of George Thomas Hospice Care

PART ONE

GROWING UP

1

The Evans family background

I WAS BORN on 30 May 1932 in Aberystwyth, the elder son of the Rev. Dan Evans, born 1887, the minister of Siloh Chapel in the town. It was one of the largest Welsh churches within the Presbyterian Church of Wales, known originally as Calvinistic Methodists and referred to in Welsh as *Yr Hen Gorff*. My mother, Mary Ann Williams, born 1892, was a farmer's daughter to Morgan and Margaret Williams, Glanrhyd, Cilycwm, near Llandovery. They were married in Soar Chapel, Tŷ Newydd, Cilycwm on 9 August 1919.

They had five children who survived into adulthood. Mair, born 1925, was head girl at Ardwyn Grammar School, Aberystwyth in 1942 and trained as a nurse at University College Hospital, London where she met and subsequently married Dr John Turner who practised as a GP in Llanidloes, Bargoed and Tregaron before retiring to Aberystwyth – Mair died in 2004 and John in 2007. Enid, born 1928, left Ardwyn Grammar School at an early age to look after the family while my mother was hospitalised for a period. This was a great sacrifice for which we are indebted to her. She married Derrick Pryse, and emigrated to Australia where she now lives in Perth and is a very fit 84 year-old – Derrick died in 2000. Rhiannon, born 1930, died the day after I was born. Mother referred to her as 'God's chosen one'. Trefor, born 1933, is my brother by 15½ months. He married Ann Davies and they now live in Llandybie after a successful and varied career as a chartered accountant – he had a successful practice in north Carmarthenshire, the home area of both parents. Ann, born 1939, the youngest sister, trained as a nurse at Llandough Hospital, Cardiff, and joined the Queen Alexandra's Royal Army Nursing Corp (QARANC). She married Brian Macdonald, emigrated to Australia and they now live in Melbourne. We were known in Aberystwyth as 'Dan Evans Siloh's children'.

My father had an interesting background. The birth certificate records that he was born at Wernpwll, Rhandirmwyn to John Evans, a lead miner who signed the birth certificate with X and Rachel Evans (formerly Morgans), a domestic servant. He was brought up by a single parent mother. He felt called to the Christian ministry at a young age, started preaching soon after the 1904/5 Revival in Wales, then studied at a school in Carmarthen before going to Trefecca and then to University College, Cardiff, obtaining a BA degree. He continued further studies at the Theological College, Aberystwyth. His studies were interrupted by the First World War during which he served for 3½ years in Mesopotamia with the Royal Army Medical Corps (RAMC).

Before coming to Siloh, Aberystwyth where he served for over 25 years from 1925 to 1951, he was minister of Siloh, Llanelli (1919–23) and then Bethlehem, Porth, Rhondda (1923–5). My parents moved from Aberystwyth to Llandybie in 1951, to care for two small churches – Gosen, Llandybie and Tirydail, Ammanford (1951–8). They retired to Llandovery in 1958, where my father continued to preach every Sunday until his admission to Llandough Hospital, Cardiff, where he died on 9 February 1962 aged 74 years. He left written instructions for a private cremation funeral, no flowers, and donations to the Foreign Mission.

After my father's death in 1962, my mother found it very hard to cope and came to live with the family in Cardiff but found it difficult to settle. She spent some time in Northern Ireland before returning to live with Edwina and myself then, having never travelled further than London, went to visit Enid and Derrick in Australia, after which she returned to us. We were by then living in Shepperton, London. Mother declared that she wanted to live in Wales, so she moved to Aberystwyth for a while before finally settling in a convalescence home in Lampeter, where she was very well cared for in a Welsh setting. After a prolonged, painful and distressing time she died at Priory Street Hospital, Carmarthen on 4 July 1975, aged 82 years. Sadly, during those 13 years after father's death she suffered heart failure and was resuscitated twice, although her wish was to join her beloved husband in heaven with the Lord. In later years I stated publicly, as a committed Christian, my opposition to euthanasia/assisted suicide and also pleaded for a reappraisal of the medical policy of preserving life at all costs. I've warmly welcomed the revised guidance by the General Medical Council, 'Treatment and care towards the end of life; good practice in decision making' which came into force on 1 July 2010. I'd been asked, as the elder son, following my father's admission to Llandough Hospital in 1962, if they could operate to prolong his life for a short while. I refused saying "please let my father die in peace" and I have always had a clear conscience regarding that decision.

Having experienced the responsibilities and demands of leading churches as an elder in later years I was amazed at my father's ability to cope with such a heavy workload. He had pastoral care of some 800 members plus visitors and students, preaching at least twice on Sundays – to my knowledge he never preached the same sermon twice at his home church – leading the midweek meetings, preaching throughout Wales and in London and Liverpool, and sitting on various committees. The concept of a team ministry was alien in those days!

My father was a big man, both physically and spiritually. He spent many hours alone in his study in preparation. The *Cambrian News* kept him supplied with free offset note paper on which he would write his sermons. He made Trefor and me promise to burn his sermons after his death which we dutifully did in Llandovery the day after his cremation. It was quite a bonfire, representing over 50 years of preaching ministry. Sadly, I've forgotten most of my father's sermons but remember clearly him emphasising that the true Christian life was at odds with the ways of the world and adding 'if you go against the grain you can expect to collect splinters'!

A key to my father's lifestyle was that he managed time well and I recall, as a teenager, being advised that one of the most important lessons in life was to be disciplined about the use of time. This aspect is best illustrated by the use of his trusty pushbike, a heavyweight model befitting a 6 ft-plus man, when doing pastoral visiting. It had the prime benefit of flexibility and low cost so that when he saw a member or colleague he would dismount for a quick chat. He never had a car.

In addition to his workload my father was Moderator of the Presbyterian Church in Wales in 1958. The following extract from his appeal to the Connexion to support the Home Mission (Forward Movement) reflected his core beliefs and priorities as a minister of the gospel:

> The early Church came to a pagan world and saved it from dying. The Church today lives in a society that is becoming more and more pagan. There are many factors in the paganism of today but the results will be the same, destruction and death. We rejoice that life has become easier for our people, but like that farmer in the parable, we may feel secure with our earthly possessions and lose our souls in the bargain. And what shall it profit us to gain the whole world and lose our very souls?

He warned me, shortly before his death that the spiritual situation would become darker unless there was another God-given Revival in Wales.

My parents were strong characters – father with a positive personality while mother was strong-willed and dominant. Father was head of the family but mother was clearly in charge of running the home. It really was a happy marriage and they were a great team. Father maintained the same Christian principles and practice in the home as in the pulpit, while mother was essentially a practical housewife – an excellent cook she would turn out tarts, jam sandwiches and Welsh cakes by the dozen. She was very house-proud, believing that cleanliness was next to godliness!

The manse, Beth Seilun, was built between Siloh Chapel and Savage's Garage in Queen's Road, Aberystwyth was a substantial house and my parents and youngest sister Ann lived there until we moved to Llandybie in 1951. Siloh Chapel, built 1863, has now been demolished. The vestry built behind the manse and the ground floor of Beth Seilun have, since 2005, been linked and developed as a community facility renamed Morlan, while the first and second floors continue as residential accommodation. The emergence of Morlan as a community facility has thrilled me because it mirrors the development of a community centre and church I was involved in as an elder in Thornhill, Cardiff.

When I was leaving home for the first time in 1949 (to work at Barclays Bank, Newport, Shropshire) my father gave me a special verse, in Welsh, to remember daily – Psalm 51 v.10: 'Crea galon lân ynof, O Dduw, ac adnewydda ysbryd uniawn o'm mewn.' ['Create in me a pure heart, O God, and renew a steadfast spirit within me.' (NIV)] It was fulfilled 16 years later in Ashford, Middlesex.

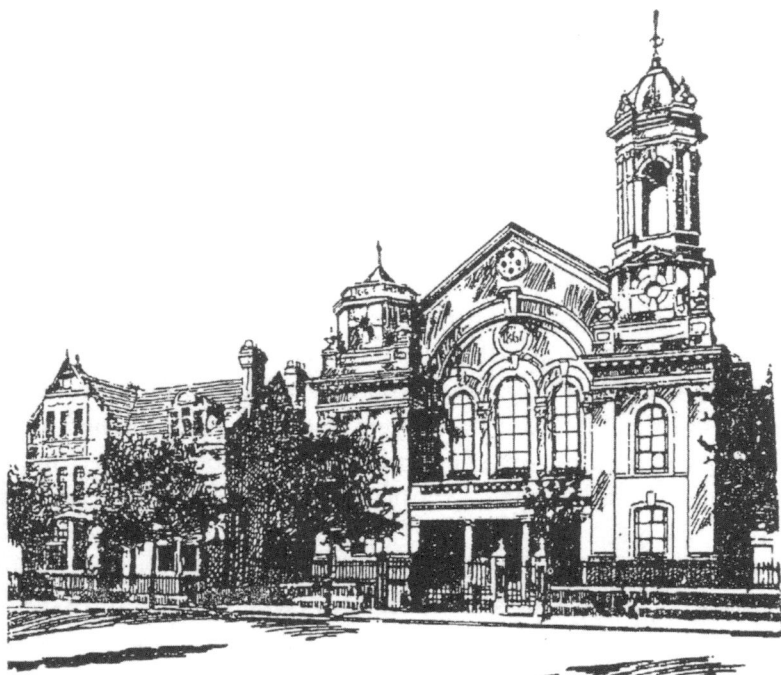

Siloh Chapel and Beth Seilun (the Manse), Aberystwyth

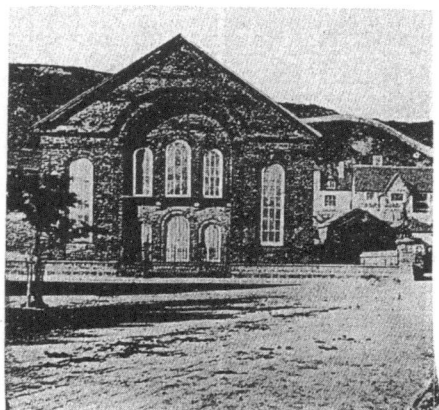

1863

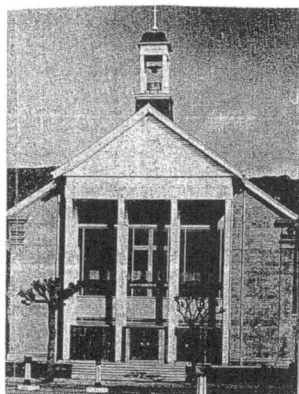

1963

2

The early years in Aberystwyth

DESPITE ALL THE pressures on our parents, the Evans children enjoyed a happy childhood with Welsh the language of the home. As children we were encouraged to develop our own personalities but were firmly reprimanded if we misbehaved. Trefor was a more robust character than me but, when trouble was afoot, I was held to blame as the older one who should know better!

Many memories come flooding back from those early childhood years. One such memory is when Trefor and I were allowed to attend for the first time the afternoon session of the Gymanfa Ganu at Siloh Chapel. We sat in the front row of the gallery, behind the clock facing the pulpit. Trefor was that small he could barely see over the balcony. The chapel was full and capable of seating about 1,000, but when the singing gave way to the chairman's address, we lost interest and started to explore the workings of the clock. Suddenly, the chairman's remarks stopped mid-sentence with the comment "I've seen that clock move half an hour while speaking"! We were taken home without further ado.

On another occasion, we hid behind the coal house with a bottle of non-alcoholic communion wine which was kept in the pantry for use on pastoral visits. We rather liked the taste but realised to our horror that we had drunk most of the contents. We managed, without being discovered, to top it up with Ribena!

Apparently I would not go to school at the compulsory age of five without Trefor attending too, so we started at

Alexandria Road Board School, Aberystwyth together. One day, to our shame and embarrassment, we were disciplined for having shut some girls in the toilets and had to stand in the corner before the class. My comment was "I don't like this school" to which Trefor replied "We'll burn it down when I grow up"!

The only occasion our father exercised physical punishment, fully justified, was when we climbed on to the roof of the chapel via Savage's Garage and the vestry. We knew from his "Boys, come down at once" (in Welsh) that we were in big trouble, so took time descending and crept up behind him in the backyard – he was, of course, fearful that we might fall. Without further ado, he ordered us into the back kitchen to receive a gentle slap on bare bottoms – me first and then Trefor, who had already pulled down his trousers ready for the punishment. My mother told me years later that father had a job to keep a straight face!

I recall clearly when Trefor and I had our tonsils removed at the local hospital, Aberystwyth General. Trefor, who went down to theatre first, hit out at the chloroform anaesthetic which explained why when my turn came, I found myself pinned down on the theatre table.

Our playtime was robust. Trefor broke my forearm while playing submarines by tossing me over the back of an armchair with the words "it's your turn to be a diver".

As we grew up, we became more adventurous, with Cwm Woods, the Buarth, Constitution Hill and the rocks below becoming our playground. Unlike today's generation, we developed our own leisure activities.

It was normal to attend chapel services on Sunday morning and evening and Sunday school in the afternoon, and Band of Hope one evening during the week. In later years, I would accompany my father to the midweek seiat/prayer meeting. On one very embarrassing occasion my father asked me to choose a hymn to close the meeting and I gave out a hymn that had been sung earlier in the meeting!

There were also special meetings involving the denomination's foreign mission field in India and these made a big impression on me – lantern slides of the work and little yellow boxes for saving pennies as gifts towards the work overseas.

Many visitors called at Beth Seilun. I remember being introduced to Dr Martyn Lloyd-Jones (then minister of Westminster Chapel, London) when he preached at Siloh. Another frequent visitor who made an abiding impression was Rev. Nantlais Williams from Bethany, Ammanford and the editor of *Trysorfa'r Plant*, a monthly magazine in Welsh for children.

On one particular Sunday morning it was a children's service, and a group of boys, including me, aged 10/11 were to sing two verses of a hymn they had learnt at Sunday school. It was a disaster. The boys stood on a dais behind the organ facing Mr Charles Clements, a renowned organist, and the congregation. Mr Clements' facial expression changed as we started to sing out of tune. It got worse, so the organ drowned our voices for the second verse – leaving our Sunday school teacher in tears. The boys never participated again as a group.

I had the temerity once to suggest to my father over Sunday lunch that one of his members fell asleep during the sermon – only to be admonished with the comment that "that member memorises the whole sermon and we discuss the contents midweek". There was one elderly church member who made a lasting impression, namely, John Evans. He and his wife were dependant on deaf aides during the Sunday services. At the midweek meetings he would read the Scriptures and pray on his knees with passion. Apparently, in his younger days, he was a blaggard, blasphemer and a wife beater, before conversion in the 1904/5 Revival.

Before the outbreak of the Second World War in 1939, my family would spend August in our mother's old home at Glanrhyd, Cilycwm. The land was being farmed by a neighbour, Dan 'Ochrfforest'. It was a wonderful holiday home with the house located only a few yards from the banks of the River Towy. We would decamp from Aberystwyth with the help of a Potts removal van with father acting as navigator, and the rest of the family following in a taxi. At the bottom of the garden in Glanrhyd were the ruins of the original farmhouse in a state of collapse but with the staircase giving access to a bedroom where Trefor and I discovered an old army cap hanging on the wall. We decided to collect as many eggs as possible from around the farm and see who could hit the soldier's cap with an egg thrown from the other side of the room. Our misdemeanour (call it original sin!) came to light when Dan Ochrfforest complained that there were no eggs to be found. He was, of course, compensated for the loss. On many occasions, when we played cricket between the chapel and Beth Seilun, our father bore the cost of broken windows.

One very painful experience remains of those halcyon holidays at Glanrhyd. It was the first occasion that we had seen an aeroplane in the sky, and decided to replicate it by folding a page of the *Western Mail* into a paper model. To ease out the creases, we decided to put it through the large wooden mangle – Trefor turning the handle while I inserted the nose of the plane between the rollers. Unfortunately, the top of my three middle fingers were crushed in the process. The screams could be heard in Rhydfelin some ¼ mile away – they thought a pig had been slaughtered!

I would often accompany my father when he visited his mother at Brynfforest just up the hill from Rhydfelin. A big attraction was one of those original gramophones with a huge loudspeaker – wound by hand with music on wax cylinders.

Christmas time at Beth Seilun was always a joyful family time. The goose was supplied from Clynmawr Farm, near Cilycwm. It would be put on the bus at Llanwrda and collected at Aberystwyth. On one occasion we accompanied father to meet the bus and collect the goose, but the conductor and driver assured them that no parcel had been handed in on the bus journey from Ammanford. Back to Beth Seilun and mother swooned on hearing the news: 'dim gwydd' [no goose]! Then the doorbell rang with a telegram saying 'missed bus – parcel tomorrow' which was received with great relief. Home-made Christmas pudding was another treat, with us searching for the groat hidden within. Us children would decorate the kitchen with hand-made decorations, and put on a mini concert for our parents using the large dining table as a stage. Oh happy days!

There were other incidents during childhood in Aberystwyth which made the national news. We remember being taken by our father to see the extensive damage caused by a sea storm in January 1938 which washed away the end of the pier and a large stretch of the promenade near Alexandra Hall, a residence for students.

We also remember King George VI and Queen Elizabeth passing Beth Seilun on their way to open the extension to the National Library of Wales on Penglais Hill in 1937. My father was involved as the Chaplain to the Mayor of Aberystwyth.

3

Wartime memories

THE SECOND WORLD War brought major changes and some very sad memories. The hotels and guest houses in Aberystwyth were requisitioned for military personnel undergoing square-bashing on the promenade. Enemy planes flew overhead at night to bomb Liverpool. We accommodated two evacuees from Liverpool for a short while. They were promptly fed and bathed on arrival in Beth Seilun until their skins were pink! The following morning Trefor and I took them for a walk on the promenade. Apparently, they had never seen the sea before and one nearly drowned when he ran down the slipway into oncoming waves.

Another haunting memory was of a column of bedraggled soldiers, rescued from Dunkirk, winding its way down Queen's Road, Aberystwyth – with each household being asked if they had a spare bed or room. Trefor and I were playing in front of Beth Seilun and volunteered, without consulting with our parents, to take in two soldiers as there was a spare bedroom on the second floor. What a culture shock for them. I can remember them having to stand in the back yard waiting entry to the house while my mother washed the hallway and waited for it to dry, before she would allow them entry!

It was wartime and the whole family had individual ration books. It was decided to allocate each of the seven ration books to seven separate grocery shops in the town where a church member worked or was the owner. One of my tasks on a Saturday morning would be to visit each shop in turn and collect one's allocation for the week. The contents were so meagre, but we seemed all the healthier for it.

One other aspect of family life at that time was that everyone would gather for supper at 8.55 p.m. – in time to say grace and listen to the 9 p.m. news on the radio. After supper, my father would return to his study on the first floor while we had designated tasks to undertake before bedtime. My task was cleaning and polishing the family footwear. I was also responsible, usually on a Saturday morning, for sweeping the back yard and cleaning the windows on the ground floor of Beth Seilun. These skills have never left me.

4

Escape to the farm – Nantiwrch, Caio, Carmarthenshire

WITH THE OUTBREAK of war, I started taking holidays on my uncle's hill farm, Nantiwrch, near Caio, where I spent some of the happiest days of adolescent life. I would travel by bus from Aberystwyth, alight at Maestwynog and walk the 2½ miles or so to the farm. Life was so different there – enriching and educational. The food, all home produced, was tasty and nourishing. Initially, I slept in a double bed on a feather mattress between my two adult cousins Dai John and Sam Davies, both 6ft 5in tall. Later DJ, a gifted craftsman and poet, left the farm to become one of the first employees of Dr Iorwerth Peate at St Fagans Folk Museum in Cardiff. Within a year or two, I had become a useful farm hand, driving the tractor while cousin Sam would be on the hay machine or binder. In addition to Nantiwrch, they also farmed Garreg in Caio.

It was an idyllic life. The farmers in the neighbourhood helped each other at times of hay-making, harvesting, sheep shearing and sheep dipping. That community life has long since disappeared through increased mechanization, merging of farms and greater emphasis on stock rearing. Sam's grandson Aled now farms Nantiwrch single-handed. I learnt the art of milking but the cows realized I was a novice and only yielded about 50 per cent of the contents of their udder for me! One of my tasks was to separate the milk, so that the calves could be fed and the cream retained for churning into butter.

The area had a rich cultural tradition. Each community held an annual eisteddfod usually in a local chapel or village hall. Cousin DJ was a gifted poet and a regular competitor. He took me to my first eisteddfod held in Siloh, a small hamlet between Maestwynog and Llandovery. It was a warm day and the chapel was packed to overflowing. DJ had arranged for me to collect the prize if the nom-de-plume 'Y boi bach' [The little boy] was declared the winner. And so it was following the adjudication, that I went forward to collect the prize from the chairman, who was the local minister, only to be asked was I the author of the poem? No, I cried pointing to DJ, standing at the back, to everyone else's amusement.

In those days, there were rabbits aplenty, before myxomatosis, and they ravaged young crops. Cousin Sam was a keen trapper and allowed me to accompany him, after supper, to collect those caught on condition I helped to gut them. Many a night we would return with some thirty rabbits for gutting in the barn. Initially I would retch but soon acquired the skill of cleaning out the innards in one fast action. It was wartime and fresh meat was scarce. Rabbits were much sought after and were taken to Swansea market and sold, providing a useful source of income.

Another highlight was attending the markets in Lampeter, Llandovery or Carmarthen. On one occasion, at Lampeter, I arranged to meet Sam around the sale ring after buying an ice cream. On returning to the market I spotted Sam on the opposite side and endeavoured to catch his attention by raising an arm. But every time I did so, the auctioneer apparently took it as a bid and the price of the animal in the ring went up!

In those wartime days, all farmers had to submit records to the Ministry of Agriculture of activities on the farm – 'Dig for Victory' was the nation's motto. The information provided was often checked by visits from inspectors and were the basis for paying subsidies. I would compile these returns under Sam's guidance and deliver them personally to the Ministry of Agriculture office in Carmarthen – now the iconic building and headquarters of Carmarthenshire County Council overlooking the River Towy.

One unforgettable character from that period was Dan 'Erw-Domi', a small holding near Nantiwrch. He was a large rotund figure who kept his paper money wrinkled up in little balls. Dan would always arrive for any co-operative activity, e.g. sheep shearing, in time for lunch, tea or supper. I have never laughed so much as when Dan would be instructing his dogs to gather stray animals – he expected the dogs to do the impossible!

Nantiwrch kept two horses and a pony. One day when I was about 13 years old I went, by pony, to Caio to collect some provisions from the village shop/post office. Not having fully mastered the art of pony riding, I took my time for the three-mile journey and, having filled the rucksack with sugar, and prunes etc., slowly made my way up the very steep hill out of the village towards Nantiwrch. Once over the brow I decided to quicken the pace and found it more comfortable galloping than trotting. A neighbouring farmer, who happened to witness the scene, claimed later, "Adrian rode like a jockey winning the Derby"! Arriving back in Nantiwrch and feeling rather pleased with myself, I was confronted by Uncle (a man of very few words) who, looking at the pony belching steam and dripping with perspiration, cried "Have you tried to kill the little pony?" Worse was to follow – the individual bags of sugar, flour and prunes had split in the rucksack – with inevitable consequences.

One further incident, which had far-reaching consequences for good, occurred when I was 16 years old and, by now, was a fully-fledged farm worker and earning my keep. It was a visit by an elderly Aunty Pugh from London with her son John who had spent holidays at the farm when a teenager. Cousin John had trained as a doctor at UCH, London and, because of indifferent health, had emigrated to South Africa where he was an ENT specialist. They were about to leave

Nantiwrch after an enjoyable day reminiscing about old times with Aunty Pugh and Uncle agreeing what a great chap Lloyd George was, when I plucked up courage to ask cousin John to examine my ears which were painful. As requested, John peered into my ears with the aid of a torch and felt behind the ears. When I confirmed that I'd suffered earache for years, especially after swimming, John immediately went back into the farmhouse and wrote two letters – one for the family doctor and the other for a chemist in Aberystwyth. I returned home to Aberystwyth the following day with the letter to the family doctor requesting that I be seen urgently by an ENT Specialist in either Cardiff, London or Edinburgh. The letter to the chemist was for a new drug which proved unavailable at that time in the UK, though it was in use in South Africa and USA.

The outcome was that I was seen by Mr Robert Owen in Cardiff, spent three months in the Charles Radcliffe Ward at Cardiff Royal Infirmary having major radical mastoid surgery on both ears and nose. I became a trusted patient, helping the nurses pack gauze dressings into drums for sterilizing – there was no Central Sterile Services Department (CSSD) or disposable dressings in 1947. On my discharge from the CRI, I thanked Mr Robert Owen but asked why was I still partially deaf. Mr Owen's reply was "My boy, you are fortunate to be alive"!

5

Happy Memories of Ardwyn Grammar School, Aberystwyth (1943–9)

(Extract from the Ardwynian Association Newsletter No. 40, May 2010)

I ENJOYED NON-ACADEMIC activities more than studying but did manage to gain a school certificate of matriculation standard. It took me an extra year because of a three-month hospital stay for major ear surgery in 1947.

It was a great privilege to play for the school: fly-half at rugby, goalkeeper in soccer and as an all-rounder in cricket. The annual First XV versus the local public schoolboys and the hockey match against the girls' team are still vivid memories.

Other highlights were taking part in the Gilbert & Sullivan and other operas in the King's Hall at the end of the autumn term. I played the Queen's Fool in *Merrie England* and in the Welsh drama night at the end of the spring term. The opera soiree was another enjoyable event.

As a prefect I acted as captain of the rowing club and had to ensure that before setting out to sea in the school boat, the permission of the kindly Capt Lewis, Portland Road had been obtained.

An activity which served us well in later life was the

lunchtime dancing class in the gym and the end-of-term dance in the school hall was the catalyst for so many boy/girl relationships as well as the opportunity to scrump apples from the school garden. This activity caused the cancellation of these evening dances for a period.

School dinners in the hall have special memories too – sitting on benches seven or eight each side of trestle tables. Some played push penny football culminating in a cup final at end of term.

The debating society was another enriching experience with a mock election the highlight. Distinguished fellow pupils were John Morris, then an ardent Liberal and subsequently Labour MP for Aberavon, QC, Secretary of State for Wales and Attorney General; and Elystan Morgan, then a fiery Welsh Nationalist, later Labour member for his native county Ceredigion, judge and member of the House of Lords. I stood as an Independent, coming third after Elystan and John (now respectively Lord Elystan Morgan and Lord Morris of Aberavon).

There was great excitement when the mixed choir, trained by music and woodwork teacher Mr Roberts, travelled to Carmarthen to record a programme for the BBC.

Of the staff, I appreciated the far-sightedness of headmaster Mr D C Lewis who developed in us a pride and ethos for the school. I'm grateful also to Mr Lloyd, chemistry, and Mr Roy James for inculcating their love of rugby and cricket to us youngsters.

Initially, I failed to take the advice of careers' master Mr Sam Mitchell, and I joined Barclays Bank. After six months, recurring ear problems and increasing deafness caused me to leave the bank and take a temporary clerical post at Aberystwyth General Hospital. This led to a career in the National Health Service retiring early in 1983 as the chief administrator and secretary of the South Glamorgan Health Authority.

6

My wife Edwina and mother of Trefor and Huw

I FIRST MET Edwina at a roll-a-penny stall in a funfair at Machynlleth – she was a student nurse at Guy's Hospital, London and was home on holidays. I was at that time secretary of Machynlleth Chest, Machynlleth and District, and Towyn Memorial hospitals.

Edwina was born in Islington, London on 4 July 1932 but grew up in Machynlleth – one of four children to Mary Winifred Lane Hughes. They lived with Edwina's grandfather, David Hughes, at 108 Maesgwyn Street, a house which had been built in 1628. David Hughes was huntsman to the Plas Machynlleth Foxhounds until he retired in 1933.

Edwina's mother worked initially as a school dinner lady and later as cook at the Chest Hospital, Machynlleth. After retirement, she moved to sheltered accommodation in Newtown before moving to Cardiff to live with Edwina and myself for the latter years of her life. Although nearly blind she was an avid follower of snooker on TV. She died peacefully, her childhood Christian faith restored, on 28 April 1987, aged 83 years.

Edwina worshipped in the Church in Wales, and attended the elementary school and then the county school in Machynlleth. She excelled in sport and still, at 80 years of age, loves watching tennis on TV. She left home at the age of 18 and spent five years in London nursing at the Samaritan Free Hospital for Women and Guy's Hospital. The highlight of those years was waiting all night on the Mall to see the coronation of the Queen in 1953. Her final year as a staff nurse at Guy's was spent to qualify for her Guy's badge. I had already moved into a top-floor flat in Connaught Road, Cardiff and that year of separation cost us a fortune in communication.

We were married on 1 March 1956 in Siloh Chapel, Aberystwyth, with my father, the Rev. Dan Evans officiating. We travelled by train to Stratford-upon-Avon for our honeymoon. At Welshpool station, I dashed to the station buffet to get two cups of tea only to see the train starting to move without me and Edwina gesticulating wildly from the carriage window. A further embarrassment occurred when I forgot to sign her in at the White Swan Hotel, Stratford. We were blissfully happy in the flat in Connaught Road despite having to stuff numerous copies of the daily newspaper behind skirting boards to prevent draughts during the winter time.

Edwina worked part-time as a staff nurse at Rhydlafar Orthopaedic Hospital from 1956–9. After caring for the children she returned to part-time work as the school nurse at Cardiff High School from 1975–90.

Trefor, our eldest son, was born on 17 June 1959 and is now a director of a large international construction firm specializing in project management in Bristol. He obtained his degree at Swansea University and is qualified both as a chartered civil engineer and as a chartered structural engineer. He married Jill Rose Harding at Grove Chapel, Camberwell, London on 29 March 1986. She had qualified as a primary school teacher at Cambridge University. They have two sons – Joe born 1990 in Romania and adopted when a baby, and Olly born in Cardiff in 1996.

Huw, our second son, was born on 15 June 1963 with spina bifida and hydrocephalus, and his life is a case study of the remarkable progress made in medicine during the past 50 years. A breakthrough occurred when an American engineer developed a one-way valve which relieved pressure on the brain. It so happened, when Huw was born, that a senior registrar in neurosurgery at Cardiff Royal Infirmary (where I was working at the time) had worked in Sheffield – one of the pioneering centres in the UK for spina bifida cases. He inserted a spitzholter valve when Huw was a week old – it is still there after 48 years. The surgeon was reluctant to operate because of the extensive open lesions on Huw's spine – he is paraplegic from the waist – but there was no other option as he faced death. He was christened and committed to the Lord by Uncle Daniel, only brother of my mother, Rev. D J Williams, minister of Salem Presbyterian Church, Canton, Cardiff where Edwina and I were members. Huw survived, as he has done on at least six other occasions when his life has been spared. He has overcome his disabilities remarkably well and lives independently in a bungalow adapted for his needs.

Huw started his education in a school for the handicapped in Hounslow, Middlesex. At the age of nine he was chosen for the *Magpie* appeal, an ITV children's programme, for spina bifida children and raised a record sum of £79,000 in 1973. Having later entered mainstream education and passed his driving test with a motability scheme car, he attained GCE O levels, a BEC National Certificate in business studies in Coventry and finally a degree in law at the University of Glamorgan. He went to work in the tax office at Llanishen, Cardiff for 13 years before being medically retired. Huw is now self-employed, owning and renting houses in Cardiff to students – the entrepreneur of the family and an inspiration to all. As a family, our lives have been so enriched through him, not least in his acquisition of culinary skills in later years and providing his parents with superb meals.

One final memory. Following Trefor's birth in 1959 we vacated the flat and bought our first house in Lakeside, Cardiff by selling the A35 car and using the £250 as a deposit – 10 per cent of the mortgage on a three-bed semi. How times have changed!

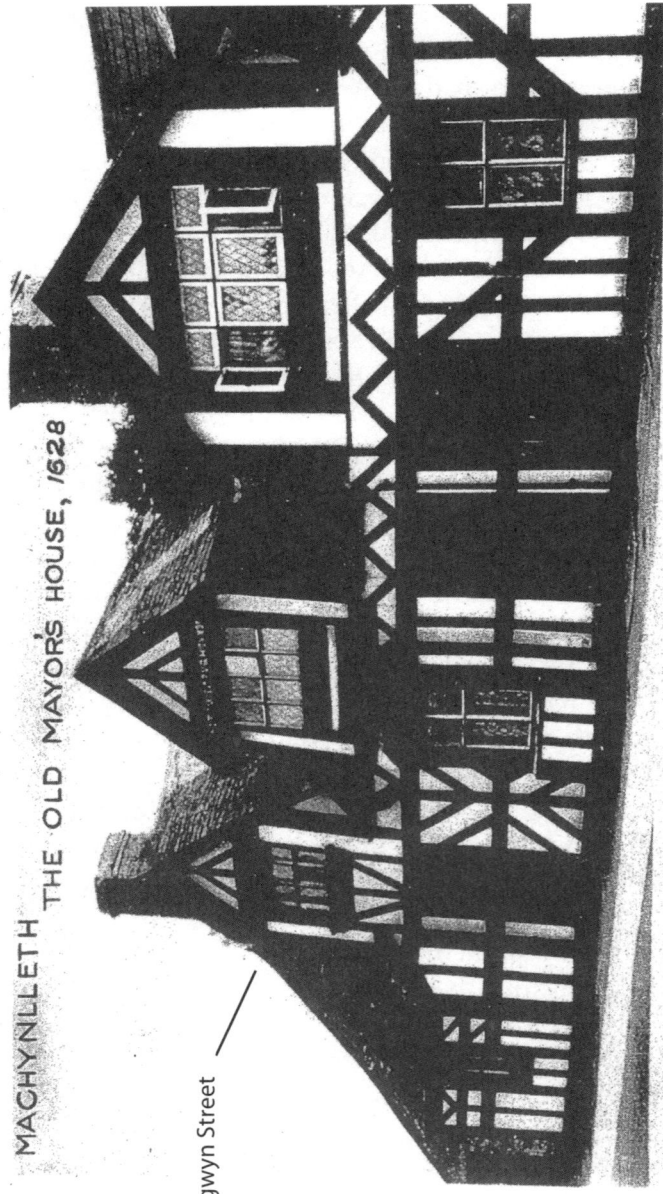

MACHYNLLETH THE OLD MAYORS' HOUSE, 1628

IN THE OLDEN TIMES THE MOST IMPORTANT OFFICES IN MID-WALES—TRANSACTING THE MANORAL RIGHTS OF CYFEILIOG AND ARWYSTLI; AND THE CHARTERED POWERS OF THE OLD CORPORATION OF MACHYNLLETH. THEY WERE TAKEN BY CROMWELL'S YEOMANRY, UNDER SIR THOMAS MIDDLETON, EARLY IN NOVEMBER, 1644.—E.J.

108 Maengwyn Street

PART TWO

WORKING IN THE NATIONAL HEALTH SERVICE

7

The start of a career in mid Wales (1950–4)

My first job in the NHS was in a temporary clerical post at Aberystwyth General Hospital, setting up a stores' control system. The appointment was made permanent and I was allocated to the finance department of the mid Wales Hospital Management Committee (HMC). The HMC had been formed, under the NHS Act 1946, to administer a group of hospitals in mid Wales, with effect from 5 July 1948.

The creation of the NHS was a towering and monumental achievement by Aneurin Bevan, who was responsible for health in the post-war Labour Government. In implementing his scheme he had to concede the right to private practice in order to gain the support of the medical profession including a system of merit awards controlled by consultant medical staff themselves (a letter in *The Times*, 27 August 2010 claimed that Bevan famously said "I stuffed their mouths with gold"). The chief characteristics of health services in the UK in 1948 was a very uneven provision of healthcare, a desperate shortage of finance and a horrendous lack of investment in new hospitals and services mainly due to the war. Most of the voluntary hospitals were in financial difficulties and many local authorities had failed over the decades to build new hospitals. The Middlesex County Council and Cardiff City Council were notable exceptions.

The development of a state-funded National Health Service

had been a long time coming as the following précis from the *Western Mail* indicates:

The long road towards the NHS

The idea of a state-funded health service did not emerge overnight, rather it was half a century or more in the making.

1890 – The Tredegar Medical Aid Society, which would provide Nye Bevan with the inspiration for the NHS, was born.

1920 – The Dawson Report recommended a comprehensive system under the auspices of a single authority.

1926 – The Royal Commission on National Health Insurance pioneered the idea of a publicly-funded health service.

1939-45 – The creation of the Emergency Medical Service during World War Two hastened the pace of change as this was the first time healthcare funding had been taken over by central government.

1941 – A government-commissioned independent inquiry found healthcare varied vastly across the country. Voluntary hospitals were permanently on the verge of financial collapse and the municipal hospitals were almost universally loathed.

1942 – The Beveridge Report into social care was, perhaps the final catalyst. Sir William Beveridge, an eminent economist, identified a national health service as one of three essential elements of a viable social security system.

In 1950 my working day at Aberystwyth General Hospital would start as a patient in the casualty department having my ear problems treated. What a transformation has occurred over the past 62 years in the equipment used – these days my mastoid cavity is cleaned out painlessly with magnification and suction apparatus, and there are a range of drugs to deal with infections. The contribution of the pharmaceutical industry to improving health care has been very significant indeed.

One particular incident remains in my memory from those early days. I was required to work, on a Sunday afternoon and evening, on a rota, manning the enquiry office at Aberystwyth General Hospital. It entailed working the switchboard and making sure that the admissions' book was up-to-date, in particular, that all the patients due for admission that day had arrived. By mid-afternoon that particular Sunday, all the patients had been admitted with the exception of an elderly gentleman living outside Aberaeron with a diagnosis, threatened strangulation. I swung into action – an ambulance was called and dispatched post-haste to deal with a case of attempted suicide (my interpretation). There was no answer when the ambulance arrived at the address and, fearing the worst, police were called and forced an entry. The patient was not there but was found in a nearby house waiting for transport to Aber with the diagnosis of threatened strangulation of *hernia*. It taught me a lifelong lesson about communication!

In 1952 I gained my first promotion to be hospital secretary of three small hospitals in mid Wales – the Chest Hospital & Area Chest Clinic which then served the counties of Merionethshire and Montgomeryshire at Machynlleth, Machynlleth & District Hospital, and Towyn Memorial Hospital. It was a rewarding experience, not least in meeting Edwina, my wife.

Perhaps it is often forgotten that Wales had a well-organised tuberculosis service before the NHS. A network of sanatoria and chest clinics existed throughout the Principality administered by the King Edward VII Welsh National Memorial Association (WNMA) with its headquarters at the Temple of Peace & Health in Cathays Park, Cardiff – donated by Lord David Davies of Llandinam to the Welsh nation to reflect his passion for peace (League of Nations) and health (WNMA/tuberculosis). With the absorption of the WNMA into the NHS, the Temple of Peace & Health became the headquarters of the Welsh Regional Hospital Board from 1948 to 1974 and then the HQ of the South Glamorgan Health Authority and my office from 1974 onwards.

During those years in Machynlleth there was a transformation in the treatment of TB due to new drugs, active pursuit of TB contacts and vaccination programmes and the work of the Mass Radiography Service in detecting new cases in the community. The beds in the Chest Hospital which had a full-time consultant chest physician Dr G O Thomas were increasingly filled with non-TB cases, e.g. silicosis among quarrymen, pneumoconiosis among ex-miners and farmer's lung among agricultural workers. As the patients in the Chest Hospital were mainly long-stay, I would do a regular ward round talking to individual patients regarding their stay and the non-clinical aspects of their care, e.g. catering, heating, etc. Initially, I found it puzzling that comments from patients could vary significantly even within a six-bed ward, but after these diverse views were discussed with Dr Thomas it became apparent that negative comments were often a reflection of bad clinical news, e.g. a patient's operation at Broadgreen Hospital, Liverpool had been further delayed – hence their frustration being expressed by criticism of the food. There was one particular Christmas when snow prevented me from travelling home to my parents in Llandybie. I was welcomed into Dr Thomas' home and enjoyed the best ever Christmas away from home.

The two cottage hospitals – Machynlleth & District Hospital and Towyn Memorial Hospital – served their local communities respectively, with local GPs caring for patients not needing the facilities of a general hospital in Aberystwyth. There were also visiting consultants from Aberystwyth who held outpatient clinics there and treated in-patients not requiring major surgery. The policy of the Welsh Hospital Board, endorsed by the Aberystwyth consultants was to phase out surgery in these small hospitals. This was part of a national policy as the concept of district general hospitals, such as Bronglais in Aberystwyth, gained momentum throughout the NHS. This policy was, however, put to the test in Machynlleth when one of the local GPs, Dr Lewis, periodically invited colleagues from his former teaching hospital in London to visit Machynlleth for a long weekend away from the smog of London and to treat some patients in the bargain. I was involved in these arrangements as, invariably, one of the three or four patients listed would be a private patient. It was an arrangement where everyone involved benefited. Sir Heneage Ogilvy, a London surgeon of renown came on a number of occasions and to quote a local patient's unfair quip, "If Sir HG repairs your hernia, you don't end up with a truss"!

In the broader context of ensuring high standards of care in the NHS, the increasing commitment to evaluating and monitoring standards of clinical practice in the NHS is to be welcomed – as the Bristol paediatric cardiac and the Mid Staffs Hospital inquiries have shown. This aspect of ensuring good clinical standards and dealing decisively where there are inadequate standards at individual or corporate levels is as important, in my opinion, as the millions spent to achieve a market economy within the NHS. The new system of monitoring from Summary Hospital-level Mortality Indicators (SHMI) is to be welcomed.

Another experience was being interviewed for the post of hospital secretary at the C & A Hospital, Bangor – a general hospital and the next logical step in promotion. The setting resembled a magistrate's court, with all the members and senior officers of the HMC present. A member, noting that I claimed on my CV to be a Welsh speaker, asked me to translate 'a cup of tea'. Unfortunately I replied 'dysglaid o de' as in south Walian, and not 'cwpanaid o de' in a north Wales accent I'd acquired since working in Machynlleth and Towyn. A better candidate was rightly appointed to the post, but I was beginning to learn that one of the characteristics of the Welsh was tribalism but less prominent these days, thanks to BBC, S4C, the Welsh Assembly and the Ryder Cup 2010.

On moving to Machynlleth in 1952, I acquired a James 125

motor bike which enabled me to travel between Machynlleth and Towyn, to Dole, Llandre, Derrick and my sister Enid's home before they emigrated to Australia, and to my parents' home in Llandybie at weekends (they having moved from Aberystwyth in 1951). I failed my first test in Maengwyn Street, Machynlleth by changing a right hand signal to a friendly wave of acknowledgement to a pedestrian! Some 30 years later I saw, with mixed emotions, a James 125 model in a motorbike museum in the Lake District. I later exchanged the James 125 for an old Morris 8 car – a motor bike was no fun in the depth of winter. The test for a driving licence then required an emergency stop when the examiner sitting in the front passenger seat put his hand on the dashboard. The previous owner of the car had fitted small mirrors in the top corners of the windscreen so that, when the examiner started his hand movement, I slammed on the brakes – it was on a straight stretch of road by Machynlleth Golf Club – with the examiner ending up in a heap against the windscreen – there were no safety belts in those days. I passed the test.

My love of sport continued unabated after leaving Ardwyn Grammar School in 1949. I played, when selected, for Aberystwyth RFC and joined the committee as match secretary with the responsibility of notifying all players selected for the next game. Some years later, Gwyn Martin told me that he had sought my father's permission for this because the committee met in public houses. The chairman of the club was Capt W Davies MC, a respected member of the Welsh Rugby Union who proudly claimed at a particular committee meeting that there was no other club in Wales with four doctors at the helm – Dr 'Ianto' Clifford Jones, a GP and part-time anaesthetist, and three others who had non-medical doctorates from the University of Wales: Gwyn Owens, Orville Thomas and Ivor Thomas. Carwyn James of Llanelli, Wales and British Lions fame played a few times for the Town XV, as the fly-half position in the College XV was filled by John Brace, Onllwyn's older brother.

On one particular weekend when I was staying at my parents' home in Llandybie, I was asked to play as a late replacement at fly-half for the local XV. Brother Trefor, a regular in the team, was at that time living at home and articled in Swansea and studying for his chartered accountancy qualification, having already obtained a degree at Durham University. I had a torrid game – the Llandybie scrum-half was an ex-Llanelli player with his passes so accurate and powerful. Llandybie lost largely because of my poor performance but, on leaving the field and feeling wretched, a committee member consoled me with the comment "Don't worry boy bach, you didn't understand each other's game!" That expresses the best sentiments in Welsh rugby.

Among my treasured possessions is the following letter:

ABERYSTWYTH
RUGBY FOOTBALL CLUB

President : Dr. E. D. CLIFFORD JONES

Chairman :	*Joint Secretaries :*	
Capt. W. DAVIES, M.C.	ROY JAMES	JACK GRAVELL
43 Marine Terrace	Lyndhurst, North Road	21 Northgate Street
Aberystwyth	Aberystwyth	Aberystwyth

10 October 54

Dear Adrian,

The committee have asked me to send you a word of congratulation on your promotion to the ranks of the higher bureaucracy in Cardiff. We are pleased at your social success and doubt -less, what is the club's loss will be Cardiff Club's gain. Gareth Griffiths and Alun Thomas have already lost their places, and no doubt you will now displace Bleddyn as well.

The best of luck,

Yours sincerely,

Roy James

Joint Secretary,
Aberystwyth RFC.

Adrian Evans, Esq.,
Chest Hospital,
Machynlleth.

I made no attempt to join Cardiff RFC but played for Glamorgan Wanderers – one game for the 2nd XV and many more with the 3rd, 4th, 5th and 6th XVs. With failing eyesight I finished up as a wing-forward, and my final game was against a Taffs Wells XV ending up with two black eyes and a fractured rib. I concurred with my wife Edwina – it was time to hang up the boots.

8

Part of the higher
bureaucracy in Cardiff (1954–64)

I WAS PLUCKED from mid Wales by John Phillips, then administrator of the Welsh Hospital Board's Mass Radiography Service, and appointed chief administrative assistant at its central office in Llandaff. The service operated with six mobile and three static units. The first mobile unit had been donated pre-NHS by Lord David Davies of Llandinam who was the first volunteer to have a chest X-ray – it showed he had cancer of the lungs. The responsibilities of the new post included the preparation of detailed reports on surveys carried out by the nine units, covering communities, industrial units, schools, etc. The MRS had already been partners with the Medical Research Council's epidemiology unit based at Llandough Hospital in carrying out the famous Rhondda Fach Surveys under the leadership of Professor Archie Cochran.

In 1956, following the appointment of John Phillips as training officer for the NHS in Wales, I became deputy administrator and public relations officer of the MRS with responsibilities for organising surveys and publicity throughout Wales. Not only did I get to know Wales geographically but it was a period of honing my skills for public speaking. I claimed there was nothing more demanding than appealing to some 1,000 factory workers on their lunchtime break in the canteen to have a chest X-ray for their own good. When visiting towns and villages I would appeal to the population to attend by means of a pair of loudspeakers bracketed to the roof of his car. I recall that the most receptive audience was a herd of cattle who rushed to the hedge to see what all the noise was about. This frightened the life out of me.

My years with MRS was a period of enlightenment – it brought home to me the fundamental importance of an holistic approach to health care of which hospital services were only a part, albeit the major part in terms of resources consumed. I began to realize the strategic need for a greater emphasis on prevention and health education, for early diagnosis and identifying contacts in relation to infectious disease such as tuberculosis, coupled with positive vaccination programmes. I also had an insight into the vital role of public health and other aspects of primary care services in the community. I remember a teacher telling the class in junior school that the real doctors are the men who collect our bins of waste rubbish! Not least, I saw the significance that occupational health services played – the facilities at the Port Talbot Steelworks – then employing around 13,000 – were far superior to any provision I'd seen in the NHS.

In 1959 I was seconded to the Welsh staff committee as a regional administrative trainee for higher management. The NHS had already implemented a national trainee scheme involving the King's Fund Staff College in London and Manchester University. My initial secondment took me to Newport Gwent HMC to gain experience of a large acute non-teaching hospital, Royal Gwent, and then to the board of governors of the United Cardiff Hospitals. Mr Norman Popplewell, then deputy secretary of UCH, with Dr D G Morgan, ex-medical superintendent of Llandough, the secretary, had arranged a superb programme of induction covering the teaching hospitals of Cardiff Royal Infirmary and Llandough Hospital and departments of the Welsh National School of Medicine. I quickly sensed that my enthusiasm was not matched by some of those who were to implement the programme of induction – attitudes in a minority of cases varied from indifference, "a waste of time", to "anti-admin bashing". It was a valuable lesson for, in my subsequent

45

career, I ensured that personnel undergoing training and development were tutored by people with appropriate skills and passion.

The highlight of my attachment to the United Cardiff Hospitals, indeed one of the most exciting and enriching experiences of my whole career in the NHS, was my involvement with the architectural competition for a new Medical Teaching Centre for Wales to be built on a 53-acre greenfield site, made available by the Cardiff City Council, at the Heath, Cardiff. The University Hospital of Wales was opened by Her Majesty the Queen in November 1971. The Dental Hospital and School, not part of the architectural competition, had been built and opened in 1967. The architectural competition was a unique event in the NHS and was open to all British architects. It had been agreed that, with the paucity of hospital building since pre-war days in the UK, such a large and prestigious project should not be seen as a gift to any one particular architect or group by appointment. The fees to be earned were considerable and the reputation of the successful architect/firm would be assured nationally and internationally. A distinguished panel of assessors chaired by Sir Percy Thomas, past president of RIBA, with Mr F R S Yorke and Mr J H Forshaw representing architects from the private and public sectors respectively, together with Provost A Trevor Jones, Welsh National School of Medicine, and Dr A R Culley, Welsh Board of Health, were to judge the winning design. The best design would receive a prize of £5,000, the second best £3,000 and third £2,000. A consulting engineer was in attendance in an advisory capacity to the panel. The closing date was 30 April 1960 and on that day 22 designs were deposited at Cardiff Royal Infirmary – each with a sealed envelope attached not to be opened until the assessors' report had been finalized. Unfortunately, the senior admin assistant, Miss Joan White, who had handled all the detailed arrangements under Dr D G Morgan, fell ill the day before the closing date, and I was asked to fill the gap.

It took a week to mount the designs in the Army barracks on Whitchurch Road, Cardiff, before the panel started their detailed assessment which took about a fortnight. My role was simply to look after their mundane requirements: there was a room with a telephone, a drinks' cupboard and facilities for making tea and coffee. The assessors were taken to the CRI for lunch. My lack of social skills were exposed when Mr Yorke asked for a gin and tonic, only to be given the mixture in the wrong proportions! He commented that, if not corrected he would soon be unfit to assess anything! I observed intently their deliberations and studied the various designs. There were an amazing variety of concepts presented but the overriding consideration of the winning design was the close integration of clinical areas with the academic departments of the medical school. The panel of assessors, having agreed unanimously on their choice of entries, met in Dr D G Morgan's office with the engineer advisor and me present to open the sealed envelope and identify the winning design. There was a pregnant silence – only one of the panel had even heard of S W Milburn & Partners, Sunderland, and this was followed by a bizarre sequence of events. Dr Morgan phoned Milburn with the news of their success but the call was taken by a junior architect who promptly put the phone down thinking it was a hoax by his colleague in the next office!

All the designs were then open to the public after one day reserved for the architectural press. Only about four or five representatives turned up and I was taken aback by how little time they spent studying the designs – about an hour at most on the winning design. The subsequent reviews in the architectural press were damning, even vitriolic – 'a great opportunity had been lost', the winning design was 'old fashioned' with courtyards resulting in a huge concrete building mass with multiple access at lower ground, ground and upper ground levels. I acquainted myself with the winning design in detail so that when the public, the media and especially staff who were hoping to work in 'the promised land' visited the exhibition I was able to answer their queries. It was an experience that stood me in good stead in later years.

In January 1961 another career change came with my appointment as the first work study officer in the NHS in Wales, based at the Cardiff Royal Infirmary. I was trained by ICI personnel at the King's Fund Staff College in London. The background to such an appointment arose from concern by successive governments at the escalating costs of the NHS. The fallacious belief was that, once the NHS had been established and the pool of ill-health dealt with, costs would level out. That myopic view was soon dispelled by the Gilleband Reports which acknowledged that expenditure, capital and revenue, would continue to rise with the cost of new buildings, equipment, staffing, drugs and treatments. Demographic changes and technical advances meant that the NHS would always require additional resources. Hence the introduction of work study to achieve greater efficiency and adapt best practice from industry. I remember well Mr Norman Popplewell, by then secretary to the board of governors of United Cardiff Hospitals, congratulating me on my appointment with a rider "Now I don't want any big problems"!

I chose to study the medical records department at Cardiff Royal Infirmary as its activities were at the heart of all patient services including clinical care. The study entailed analysing the workload of all outpatient clinics at CRI over a six-month period, much to the chagrin of some of the consultant medical staff who felt it an affront to their clinical independence. The study identified major factors affecting the running of clinics, viz. the number of new to old patients seen, the number of patients who came without prior appointments via their GP or the casualty department and the number who failed to keep their appointments. These were all significant factors in providing a good efficient service for patients, clinicians and staff – not least in medical records. I discussed with individual consultants their workload for each clinic, including the balance of new and old cases to be seen, and was able to adjust the number of appointments booked and make significant inroads on the waiting time for new referrals. With the involvement of a statistician from the MRC epidemiology unit at Llandough Hospital, a study was made of the age-old problem of waiting times for patients at clinics. It came to the conclusion that, the variable factors were so many, the best one could achieve was to ensure that appointment times were spread over the clinic's duration and that patients were kept fully informed if clinics were running late. Significant improvements were made within the medical records' department, and assistance to patients to find their way around the hospital by the simple expedience of painted lines on the floor: red to blood laboratory, blue to X-ray and white to physiotherapy.

During this period as work study officer there were three Evanses working in administration at the CRI – 'Educated Evans' Gary Evans who was a national trainee and an Oxford graduate – a lifelong friend who later became secretary of the Welsh Hospital Board and then chief administrator of the Gwent Health Authority, following the 1974 reorganisation of the NHS, 'Evans Above' who worked on the first floor in the finance department, and me, 'Evans the Watch' because of my work study designation. There was a fourth Evans, namely the part-time Nonconformist chaplain who was sometimes referred to as 'Evans below'!

In August 1962 I was appointed senior admin assistant, based at CRI, with responsibilities for patient services and medical staffing. Although the NHS had been in operation for some 15 years, the Ministry of Health in July 1963 called for improved communication between doctors, nurses and patients, in an effort to reorientate attitudes so that the patients' needs came first. It acknowledged that little was known objectively about patients and their reaction to treatment, and called for more consumer research and the need for increased attention to the patient's point of view. That opportunity came about when the United Cardiff Hospitals and the Welsh Hospital Board co-operated with the Social Service Department, University College, Cardiff in a sociological survey of outpatients and casualties attending the CRI, with a comparative study of the new outpatients department at Singleton Hospital, Swansea. This research, published in *The Hospital Journal* in April 1964, with me and John Wakefield, lecturer in sociology at Cardiff University as co-authors, was an eye-opener. It highlighted the enormous efforts and stress placed on patients when they were referred to a hospital outpatient clinic – affecting their relatives, transport arrangements and costs involved – only 15 per cent were aware of procedures for claiming expenses – time off work and care of other children while away etc. Sixteen per cent of patients interviewed were not satisfied with the reasons given by their GP for their referral and a third of patients did not know the name of the doctor they had seen or were to see at the outpatient clinic. Waiting times were a major problem, with a third making specific reference to the need for delays to be explained and a plea for magazines, newspapers, music and TV to ease the waiting time. Surprisingly, 90 per cent said they were satisfied with the service – an attitude confirmed in most consumer research in the NHS, illustrating the high regard and appreciation in which the service is held by the public. The survey of patients who had failed to attend clinics were revealing – one in five said they were not aware of their appointment and, of the remainder, illness or other difficulties prevented attendance, apart from 25 per cent who decided they no longer needed treatment. This failure to attend had other serious implications, not least in delaying appointments for patients on the waiting list. On a routine visit on 7 October 2010 to the ENT Clinic at the UHW, I observed the following large poster in the waiting area:

YOUR APPOINTMENT – YOUR RESPONSIBILITY
Every day in Cardiff & Vale NHS TRUST
over 200 patients do not attend their appointments

This costs your local NHS Trust £3 million per year
This means you have to wait longer to be seen
PLEASE TURN UP OR PHONE UP

One of the most tragic cases encountered by me was of a woman who died a painful death following surgery and the coroner's inquest found that the cause of death was a theatre swab left from her operation some two years earlier. She had failed to attend the clinic following that operation and no action had been taken to either make a further appointment or notify her GP, which is now done routinely if the patient has not contacted the hospital.

A third survey, of patients attending the Accident and Emergency at CRI revealed that, in the view of the hospital medical staff, seven out of ten new patients did not need hospital treatment and could have been adequately dealt with by either a GP practice or an occupational health unit. This remains a major problem in the NHS – exacerbated by the failure of primary care to provide an adequate out of hours service. However, once a patient has presented himself, a medical assessment is obligatory – failure to do so resulted in a tramp being turned away some years ago in west Wales, and he was found dead in a hedgerow 24 hours later.

Although significant improvements have been made, the NHS still has a long way to go in educating patients and staff regarding the best use of health care resources.

During this period in Cardiff, I obtained professional qualifications – membership of the Institute of Hospital Administrators in 1962 (I was elected Fellow in 1972), Institute of Work Study in 1963 and the Institute of Personnel Management in 1964 with a certificate in personnel management, with commendation, from the Welsh College of

Advanced Technology. I claim to have been a late developer, having lacked confidence to pursue a university degree on leaving school.

I'd like to record my deep appreciation to two senior colleagues who had a profound influence on my career development – Mr John Phillips, my chief at the Mass Radiography Service and later training officer for the NHS in Wales, and Mr Norman Popplewell, chief administrator of the hospitals in Cardiff prior to the 1974 reorganisation of the NHS, who emigrated to Australia to build the new Flinders Medical Teaching Hospital in Adelaide. I benefited enormously from their wise counsel, encouragement and patience.

9

A watershed experience at West Middlesex Hospital and Chiswick Maternity Hospital (1964–7)

MY DISAPPOINTMENT ON failing to obtain the post of hospital secretary at the new Glangwili General Hospital in Carmarthen was soon erased with my appointment as hospital secretary at one of the largest acute hospitals in the UK – West Middlesex Hospital in Isleworth and the Chiswick Maternity Hospital, with more than 1,000 beds serving a population of roughly 400,000. The post carried unusual responsibilities previously exercised by a medical director until his retirement, in that the hospital secretary was required to determine once an emergency admission had been accepted from the London Emergency Bed Bureau and the consultant medical/surgical team on emergency intake had all their beds occupied, where extra beds should be on other wards taking account of staffing levels. The West Middlesex worked under immense pressures with most general wards having to put up two extra beds to cope with emergency admissions especially in winter time. The hospital had a reputation of never closing its doors with the London Emergency Bed Bureau until I found that other acute hospitals to the west of London were not subjected to the same pressures. As a result, on more than one occasion I closed the West Middlesex to extra emergency admissions to the consternation of the London Emergency Bed Bureau and the North West Metropolitan Region Hospital Board.

The West Middlesex was built by the Middlesex County Council (it grew out of the Poor Law system) – the buildings were totally inadequate with some in-patients having to be taken on trolleys externally to the operating theatres. There were only six single-bed wards on the whole of the surgical block. A new medical ward block was being built to replace wards in wooden huts. An outpatient department and an accident and emergency unit were the only modern features. I had the temerity to suggest that the new medical block should be deployed for surgery with the medical beds located in the old surgical wards! The West Middlesex had major internal problems, especially staff shortages. Recruitment was difficult because of the high cost of living accommodation in the area and competition from light industry and Heathrow airport. Student nursing suffered a 30 per cent wastage and junior medical staffing was a perennial problem – they were mainly overseas graduates seeking postgraduate experience and UK qualifications but often lacking communication skills; they did not have to pass an English test in those days. I was astonished to find, on taking up the post, that all disabled visitors to in-patients were required to have written permission to park their cars within the hospital grounds, with the porter's lodge at the main gate checking and controlling the traffic. That arrangement was soon suspended as part of an open door and welcome policy towards the general public.

I recall some of the enduring memories of my turbulent and demanding experiences at West Middlesex thus.

I remember the day that Ted Dexter, the former England batsman and selector, was admitted as an emergency after being run over by his own car. It was a Saturday afternoon and the hospital switchboard rang me at home with the news that Mr Dexter had been admitted and the switchboard was overwhelmed with press enquiries. I left immediately for the hospital indicating that a press statement would be issued in an hour or so – that was my first mistake – never promise a statement before establishing the facts! On arrival at West Middlesex I found the press were there in force with one reporter having infiltrated the orthopaedic wards and was trying to recruit junior staff to keep him informed if Mr Dexter was admitted there. A press statement was issued at about 6 p.m. stating that: 'Mr Dexter, who had been admitted with severe lacerations, had been transferred to the main orthopaedic theatre for further surgery by the on-call consultant orthopaedic surgeon and that a further progress report would be issued when he was transferred from theatre.' The A&E registrar had assured me that no bones had been broken and this was conveyed to the press. At about 11 p.m. that night – the longest 5 hours ever endured – I issued a further statement, following discussion with the orthopaedic surgeon, that: 'Mr Dexter had received severe injuries including a broken leg with severe lacerations.' The press were very critical as to why the broken leg was not identified earlier but I defended the clinical decision to transfer the patient from A&E without delay and detailed examination – it is always best to be open and honest in such circumstances. Mr Dexter made a satisfactory recovery – he was given a single-bed ward and a GPO telephone extension to deal directly with personal enquiries.

At another time a petition was received from the medical mess, following my decision to dispose, with the help of the RSPCA, of the medical mess cat which, in its old age, was the subject of complaints from domestic staff. The petition, dated 18 March 1965, was headed: 'We, the undersigned, disagree strongly with the current attempt on the part of the hospital authorities to destroy the mess(y) cat.' It bore 32 signatures of all medical grades with the following additional comments:

Cats have 9 lives.

The glory is departed.

I think that the cockroaches in the kitchen should be exterminated in preference to the cat.

If he has to go, could we have a public execution of the instigator of the plot?

A fine creature.

May we have a new kitten (what at his age!!).

This cat is as fine an exhibition of pathology that ever walked on four legs (what an irrelevant remark).

I hope you do not destroy all things with pathology.

A noble animal – about the only independent creature in the hospital.

May I keep his tail?

After much persuasion – reluctantly (but please can we have a little kitten, too).

Came the day the RSPCA called, the mess cat was not to be found, but it never reappeared. Match drawn!

One of the gang involved in the Great Train Robbery was employed as a temporary theatre porter – he was a minor participant who had arranged a hiding place for the gang. He was serving his sentence in an open prison but would be able to live at home – his mother, who made the request, worked as a nursing assistant at West Middlesex – reporting regularly to the police while working for the remaining six months of his sentence. The rota for theatre porters required working alternative weekends. He arrived for work on a Monday morning in a nearly-new Jaguar car and within two days requested the weekend off to attend a party in Sheffield! Internal audit discovered, at the end of his six months attachment, that he had bribed other porters to work his shifts at weekends so that he could enjoy the high life.

The senior general surgeon at West Middlesex accused me of being responsible for the death of a patient. I had referred an emergency medical admission to the surgeon's ward late the previous night (all other general wards were coping with two extra occupied beds), but with dire consequences. The medical case had disturbed the whole ward and the surgical patient who was due for operation the following day and was of anxious disposition committed suicide by throwing himself off the second-floor fire escape. I did not harbour a guilty conscience but wished in my heart that it had not happened.

I was welcomed one day by a general physician on a ward round with the words 'I'm glad you have come to see your patient occupying one of my beds'. It came about following flooding by the River Thames in the Teddington area and the evacuation of many residents to the outpatient hall at West Middlesex. By the Saturday evening all were able to return to their homes except for one elderly gentleman who needed social care. I agreed, having been assured that Social Services would provide alternative accommodation by the following Monday morning, that he should be admitted for the weekend. But he was still there occupying a general medical bed on the following Wednesday when I visited the ward to see the consultant physician on another matter!

The consultant geriatrician asked me once to talk to an in-patient they were having difficulties communicating with because of his Welsh background. I spoke to him in Welsh and, after a few minutes, he came alive before our very eyes. It was a tragic story – the patient, who could only speak Welsh, had lived all his life in a rural village in Montgomeryshire until his wife died and then moved to his only daughter in Hounslow who had also recently died. The outcome of my involvement was to rehabilitate him to a residential home for the elderly back in Wales.

Historically, the West Middlesex claimed to have been the cradle of geriatric medicine as a specialty under the famous Dr Marjorie Warren who pioneered rehabilitation of the elderly. It was claimed that 'her patients died with their boots on'.

The West Middlesex participated from July 1965 in a major research project funded by the Ministry of Health and the King's Fund into Hospital Internal Communication (HIC). The lead researcher was Professor R W Revens who, as chief education officer of the National Coal Board, had found that a study of productivity, accident rates, sickness and turnover etc. were not dependant primarily on working conditions, ready access to coal seams, age of mine etc., but on the relationships within management, management and workers, and their ability to relate to each other and communicate on issues formally and informally. The HIC project was to test this hypothesis in hospitals. It was a very demanding exercise but richly rewarding and opened a new understanding in my mind of how organisations function. West Middlesex was one of ten hospitals participating and undertook projects as diverse as: pilot study of a paediatric and a medical ward; study of medical social work; project paper chase; enquiry into the use of operating theatres; student nurse counselling; examination of student nurse wastage; observation on a medical unit; study of patients anxieties and opinion survey of domestic services.

Two consultant physicians at West Middlesex, Drs Nelson Coghill and James S Stewart, published, in 1998, a book *The NHS Myth, Monster or Service? Action Learning in Hospitals* based on their experiences in the HIC project. The book acknowledgements include the following: 'Adrian Evans was hospital secretary at the time of the Hospital Internal Communication Project. His enthusiasm and participative style of management had a material effect on the number and quality of the studies we undertook in that project and subsequently.'

The HIC Project was the subject of on-going review by the King's Fund Hospital Centre. Professor Revens, in 1965, joined the European Association of Management Training Centres in Brussels as a research fellow. The Revens Centre for Action Learning and Research was established in 1995 at Salford University.

As part of a public relations campaign and bridge building with the local community, I invited the local press to publish a series of articles on the work of the hospital and its hopes for the future. Many overseas visitors came to West Middlesex to see and discuss how the NHS operated at local level. Among the most interesting was the head civil servant for health to the Sultan of Brunei, then reported to be the world's richest man. The Sultan had used his vast wealth to build a hospital – importing all the equipment and recruiting qualified staff from overseas. However, he was facing mounting criticism about the hospital and these pressures were exacerbated by an influx of patients from over the border in Borneo who used the hospital. In relation to the latter problem, the civil servant was taken aback when I asked if these were natives who lived in long houses – a missionary friend of mine had worked among them. I advised that the Sultan would do well, with all his wealth, to absorb this problem as the tribes involved had no healthcare facilities of any description. Regarding the other issue, the civil servant warmed to the concept of setting up a management board of worthy individuals to be responsible for the hospital and act as a barrier between the Sultan and civil servants, and the general public.

During my period at West Middlesex, our son Huw who was born with spina bifida came under the care of Westminster Children's Hospital and, as there was no conflict of interest, we joined the local branch of ASBAH – a support group for families with spina bifida. As the chairman of the group, I spent a good deal of my time explaining the many problems facing the hospital service in meeting the complex needs of spina bifida patients and their relatives. In the wider context, these patient support groups are a vital feature of the health care system – raising money for developments and research, providing an all important platform for patients and relatives and health care staff to interact to mutual benefit, and be a pressure group in the battle of priorities. I am currently a member of the Prostate Cancer Cardiff support group.

I was privileged to be a member of the joint working party appointed by the King's Fund and the Institute of Hospital Administrators. Their report 'The Shape of Hospital Management in 1980?' was published by the King's Fund in

September 1967. It was the first review of the management structure of the hospital service, although the NHS had been in existence for almost 20 years. The BMA and medical press ignored its publication!

The experience at West Middlesex proved a watershed in relation to my professional career, but a far more important change happened in 1965 to Edwina and I which was to transform our lives. It is best summed up in a modern hymn written by Rev. Vernon Higham and published as number 812 in *Christian Hymns* – the opening two lines are:

> I saw a new vision of Jesus,
> A view I'd not seen here before,

Bearing in mind my background as a son of the manse, with a fair knowledge of the Bible in Welsh, a year passed after moving to Ashford, Middlesex without Edwina or I attending any place of worship – there were so many distractions and the pressures of a new job. However, one Sunday morning, my conscience pricked me and I found myself in Ashford Congregational Church where the pastor, the late Rev. Derek Swann, was preaching. The following months brought a transformation in our lives – what had been 'head knowledge' before, thereafter became a matter too of the 'heart and soul'. The church was a vibrant, Bible believing, caring fellowship with many missionary interests, including OMF (formerly China Inland Mission started by Hudson Taylor in 1856 and now working in south-east Asia) and Christian Radio (FEBA and FEBC) which Edwina and I continue to support along with other missionary work at home and abroad.

One memory is particularly precious. Huw was undergoing surgery at Westminster Children's Hospital and the church called a special prayer meeting for us as a family. It was an unforgettable experience as the Lord calmed our anxieties and fears and granted us His 'peace that passeth all understanding'.

Our testimony, after this life-changing experience in 1965 is, 'we have trusted God in all matters and have a living relationship with a Person – the Lord Jesus Christ as our Saviour and role model, embracing the Scriptures as God's text book, and enjoyed the power of the Holy Spirit in every aspect of our lives'. Contrary to the views of Richard Dawkins and other atheists, this is no 'God delusion' but a lasting and wonderful reality – we have been recipients of God's love and amazing grace. The Bible reminds us, 'For it is by grace you have been saved, through faith – and this is not from yourselves, it is a gift of God – not by works, so that no-one can boast.' (Ephesians 2 v.8)

10

Return to Cardiff
and the premier league (1967–70)

A T THE OUTSET of the NHS in 1948, the hospitals in the Cardiff area formed three groups: the United Cardiff Hospitals (UCH) primarily Cardiff Royal Infirmary and Llandough Hospital with a board of governors accountable to the Welsh Board of Health which later became the Welsh Office; the non-teaching general hospitals including specialist hospitals such as Sully (thoracic and heart surgery) Rhydlafar (orthopaedic) and Velindre (cancer) administered by Cardiff HMC and the mental health group comprising Whitchurch (psychiatric) and Ely (mental handicap) HMC. The Cardiff HMC and the Whitchurch & Ely HMC were accountable to the Welsh Regional Hospital Board.

The post of deputy group secretary for Cardiff HMC fell vacant and I was appointed to the post in October 1967. The post had an added attraction as the group secretary, Mr Barry, was to retire in twelve months' time – he had held the post since 1948. Mr Barry and I represented the extreme ends of the spectrum in hospital administration! The first twelve months as deputy group secretary were somewhat bizarre. I had never experienced such a restful year. I was allowed out of the group headquarters in Cathedral Road once a month to visit a hospital to check the payroll and allocated tasks appropriate to a general administration grade officer. During this particular year I could probably claim to be the best read administrator in the NHS! The

Evans family, living in Llandaf, benefited – I would be home for lunch at 1.05 p.m. and for the evening by 5.05 p.m.

In September 1968 I was designated acting group secretary of Cardiff HMC – my first taste as a chief officer – hence the analogy of the Premier League. I grasped the opportunity of leadership with enthusiasm and HMC members and senior officers responded in kind. The chairman of Cardiff HMC since 1948 was Mr R G Robinson CBE JP who had been lord mayor of Cardiff. During that brief enjoyable period as acting group secretary our relationship was more akin to father and son. I recall vividly the Christmas visits around the geriatric wards – Mr Robertson and I were accompanied by the Rt Hon. George Thomas, the then MP for Cardiff West – the hospitals were within his constituency. Mr Thomas seemed to be on Christian name terms with the majority of the patients and he would always mention 'Mam', his beloved mother. A dinner in honour of Mr Robinson, to celebrate his 80th birthday, was held on 18 October 1975 – a memorable occasion with George Thomas MP, by then the deputy Speaker, the star of the evening.

I particularly enjoyed the involvement with other NHS chief officers in Wales in learning the ropes and the politics of top management. The following remain in my memory from that period.

Firstly, allocating a piece of land at the entrance of Lansdowne Hospital for the building of an area laundry and central sterile supply department. The preferred site, behind Ely Hospital, had been rejected by the planning inspector and, without an area laundry and CSSD, the University Hospital of Wales under construction could not have functioned.

Secondly, it was the practice of Mr Jeffries, the RHB treasurer, to share largesse towards the end of the financial year, and the Cardiff HMC's share was over £50,000 – in those days budgets could not be carried over to the following financial year. However Mr Jeffries rang me a week or so later saying that the special allocation had to be cut, and only half was available, to which I responded, "I'm sorry but you are too late, the equipment has already been purchased, installed and is working in the group laboratory at St David's Hospital"!

Another memory is the flooding of the Canton area and Cathedral Road when the River Taff burst its banks after prolonged rainfall – reducing all the files and paperwork of Cardiff HMC, apart from current files in use, to pulp. After the floods subsided I arranged for the lot, all stored in a substantial out-house behind the group office, to be cleared as rubbish, and to my knowledge, no enquiries were ever received regarding the missing documents!

The Cardiff HMC approved my report calling for a unified management structure for all hospitals in the Cardiff area, otherwise the new University Hospital of Wales under construction would denude existing hospitals of key staff.

Meantime, following the publication of the Ely Report, the Whitchurch & Ely HMC was dissolved by George Thomas MP, the then Secretary of State for Wales, and the medical superintendent of Ely Hospital was dismissed (he was not in good health and doing his best coping with impossible pressures). On 1 April 1969 the Cardiff & District HMC was formed with responsibility for all non-teaching hospitals in Cardiff, with its headquarters at Whitchurch Hospital. Mr D M Thomas, an elder statesman and past president of the Institute of Hospital Administrators, and a group secretary since 1948, was appointed group secretary and I the deputy group secretary of this jumbo-sized HMC.

The Ely Report into allegations of cruelty towards mentally handicapped patients at that hospital was compiled by Sir (later Lord) Geoffrey Howe QC. It was a devastating critique, although the allegations of cruelty made by an ex-employee to the *News of the World* were not upheld. The report proved a catalyst for major changes in the care of the mentally handicapped throughout the NHS. I remember visiting Ely Hospital the day after the report was published – it was a cauldron of raw emotions. Staff had been vilified in the national and local media – some were subjected to open hostility by other passengers on buses. On being taken around each ward I was emotionally drained at the sight of many of the patients and their total dependence on staff who, to their enduring credit, remained on duty despite public hostility. It was all a great shock and I felt guilty and ashamed that not once in my 20 years in the NHS had I given a thought about the care of the mentally handicapped. Such hospitals were closed institutions, isolated from local communities and the forgotten element in the NHS. A radical change of policy was embarked upon with emphasis on rehabilitation and housing as many in-patients as possible within the community (with support), but accepting that the most severe and dependant cases would always require some form of institutional care. The concept of small domestic units in the community was developed jointly with Social Services in the Cardiff area, with the management of such units resting with Social Services rather than the NHS.

From October 1967 to September 1970 I enjoyed the privilege of speaking at national and regional conferences on aspects of health care – to RHB and HMC members and chief officers, to professional associations, political parties, social services and voluntary bodies regarding changes envisaged in the Green Paper on the reorganisation of the NHS. I had increasingly realized the importance of the voluntary contribution within the NHS in all its forms, be it individual contributions, or the work of WRVS and League of Friends, or patient support groups or other charitable efforts. In a paper to the third international conference on addiction held in Cardiff in September 1970, I pleaded for this voluntary element to be given a higher priority (shades of the Big Society envisaged by Prime Minister Cameron?) and, as an example, referred to the work of the Cardiff Christian counselling group, comprising a group of individuals drawn from a number of churches who worked together to help others in need. Acknowledging the difficulties – the whole area of voluntary involvement was fraught with challenges not least the negative attitudes of some professional staff and unions – but the policy and partnership with voluntary services had to be worked on and supported to flourish.

I remember particularly my paper to a packed audience at the Reardon Smith lecture hall in Cathays Park, Cardiff on 18 April 1970 on 'Looking at the Green Paper – Reorganisation of the NHS in Wales'. I was very nervous and, to make matters worse, my front tooth had fallen out at breakfast – but the dental hospital responded in time for my appearance on stage! Soon after this conference and without much prior warning, the Secretary of State for Wales, George Thomas MP, summoned the chairman and chief officers of the Welsh Hospital Board, the board of governors of the United Cardiff Hospitals and the Cardiff & District HMC to a meeting at the Welsh Office. It proved the most effective *coup-de-grâce* I had ever witnessed. The Secretary of State was in jocular mood and, after a warm welcome to all assembled said, "I'm sure you will agree that with the building of the new University Hospital of Wales, it is in everyone's interest that there should be a unified management structure for all hospitals in Cardiff before the more fundamental reorganisation of the NHS envisaged at a later date in the Green Paper," and, turning to his permanent secretary added, "I've asked my officers to bring this about." The hospital representatives present were stunned particularly those from the teaching hospitals. On 1 October 1970 the University Hospital of Wales (Cardiff) HMC was born with Mr Norman Popplewell as chief administrator and Mr D M Thomas as associate chief. There was no room in the hierarchy for me, but that was to prove a blessing.

In 1969 I was sent on a top management course of six weeks duration at Swansea University, arranged by Harvard University's Advanced Management School of Business

Administration. I was the only NHS representative with 70 other managers drawn from industry, commerce and academia. The course had an international flavour – in addition to the faculty members and their wives from the USA, participants from Belgium, Denmark, Germany, France and South Africa were present. As the only local Welshman, I became the unofficial spokesman for the Welsh Tourist Board, and extolled the beauty of west Wales. It was an unforgettable experience – among the most rewarding aspects was the intellectual stimulation derived from mixing with such a diverse group, led by world-class input from the professorial staff of Harvard Business School and discussions based on superb case study material from real life. Surprisingly, I found much of the content such as business policy, finance, managerial accounting and control, marketing strategy and modern decision analysis of significant relevance to the NHS. I more than held my own in challenging ethical and moral aspects, or the lack of them, in takeovers, particularly the low priority given to the human costs involved. I spent the one weekend break with the family in a caravan – sleeping most of the time and recharging the batteries for the second half of the course.

During my three-year period in Cardiff, I learnt a great deal about the politics of the NHS – vested interests and the influence of party politics, despite cries that the NHS should not become a political football. The government of the day naturally wanted key appointments such as the chairmen of health authorities to be sympathetic to their policies and this was particularly so in Wales; when the Conservative government came into power after the Labour governments of the post-war era, Sir Godfrey Llewellyn, chairman of the Conservative Association in Wales, was appointed chairman of the Welsh Hospital Board. Later, with a change of government, Mr (now Lord) Gwilym Prys Davies, a distinguished solicitor but an unsuccessful Labour candidate, was appointed chairman of the Welsh

Hospital Board. The chairman of the South Glamorgan Health Authority after my early retirement in 1983 was a Conservative MP who had lost his seat in a recent election. I was also learning that the political will to make unpopular decisions such as the closure of hospitals was a distinct element in the decision making process. Furthermore, I became aware that there were warring factions within the main political parties. I recall a real flare-up at a meeting in Ely Hospital, following the publication of the Ely Report when George Thomas MP accused certain members of the Cardiff & District HMC of being 'Jim Callaghan loyalists' who were out to embarrass him over his handling of the Ely Report.

During this period in Cardiff, I served as a co-opted member of the Welsh Hospital Board's psychiatric and general hospitals advisory committee in 1969/70, was an elected member of the Welsh Council of the Institute of Hospital Administrators in 1969/70, and was a member of the Welsh Association for Social Work Development's working party on training and administration also in that year. In addition I was a member of the working party on industrial relations set up by the Welsh Hospital Board and continued as a member after moving to north-west Surrey in October 1970. I remember being asked by an 'old' Labour member of the working party how was I coping with true blue Tories in Surrey? to which I replied, "Fine, only the colour is different"!

In relation to Christian activities, following our move back to Cardiff from Ashford, Middlesex in September 1968, Edwina and I decided to worship at Heath Church, Cardiff. Sadly our uncle, Rev. D J Williams, who was the minister of Salem Presbyterian Church in Canton, Cardiff, where we had been members, had died in 1967 and, as the two boys were not Welsh speaking, the family became members of Heath Church where Rev. Vernon Higham was the minister. The church, originally built by the Presbyterian Church in

Wales's Forward Movement or the Home Mission Board, was a thriving fellowship of about 650 members and supported more than a dozen missionaries serving worldwide. To my great surprise, as a newcomer, I was appointed church secretary within a few months and continued in that role until my appointment in north-west Surrey in October 1970. Edwina and I were active in all aspects of the work and kept an open home in Llandaff, enjoying practising hospitality, including hosting a student who stayed with us during her university course. We were also, for a while, *in loco parentis* for the son of missionary parents serving overseas. Our interest in the OMF was maintained and, at one stage, I wondered if the Lord was calling me to be the administrator of the Manorom Christian Hospital in Central Thailand – a call that was subsequently answered by Andrew Jackman, then a national trainee working in the NHS in the Midlands. I became chairman of the Heath Church missionary committee and a leader of one of OMF's prayer groups in Cardiff. I also served on the OMF's regional council for the south-west region, based in Bristol.

During this period as church secretary, Heath Church decided overwhelmingly to separate from the denomination and become an independent evangelical church affiliated to the Evangelical Movement of Wales. I had no doubts about this course of action but it caused me much heartache and sadness as I had been brought up in the Presbyterian Church of Wales and my father, Rev. Dan Evans, was its Moderator in 1958. I had come to accept that the church's confession of faith and its adherence to scripture was being increasingly marginalised by the connection's liberal tendencies. There were also practical difficulties looming. With declining membership and ministers, the latter were required to preach at other churches on a rota, at presbytery level, which meant that evangelical churches would not be in control of who occupied their pulpit. We moved to north-west Surrey in October 1970 and on our return to Cardiff in

September 1973, resumed membership and I was elected an elder of Heath Evangelical Church. The church purchased the buildings from the denomination.

11

A period of testing in
north-west Surrey (1970–3)

I FELT IT was important, from a career prospect and with major reorganisation of the NHS on the horizon, to achieve a chief officer post as soon as possible. I was interviewed twice in the same week in August 1970. The first was a three-day affair for the group secretary of the East Birmingham HMC – a large and well-managed group of hospitals. By the evening of the second day, when the short-listed candidates had dinner with the chairman, I felt exhausted but, more to the point, having sat next to the chairman at the meal I realized that our attitudes and chemistry were not compatible. Following a formal interview the following day when, thankfully, I was not appointed, I travelled from Birmingham to Surrey. Following a two-day interview, I was appointed group secretary with the title of chief executive officer to the North-West Surrey Group HMC – at least with the designation of CEO I knew where the buck stopped. It was a very large diverse group of hospitals following an amalgamation of three HMCs – a general group with St Peter's Hospital, Chertsey as the district general hospital, Botley's Park (mental handicap) and Holloway Sanatorium (psychiatric) in Virginia Waters. The chairman of the North-West Surrey Group was a practising solicitor and among the HMC members was the wife of an attorney general and the wife of the local MP – all true blue Conservatives.

Initially, we lived in temporary accommodation in New

Ham, in a house acquired for the proposed M25 motorway route. My mother and Edwina's mother had come to live with us for a while – six in a four-bedroom house was a bit demanding but grace prevailed. Edwina's mother returned to sheltered accommodation in Newtown, mid Wales where Edwina's sister was nursing. My mother, who had returned from a visit to Australia, wanted to live in a Welsh environment, so moved to Aberystwyth and later to a residential home in Lampeter. In the meantime, we purchased a new home in a small development in Upper Halliford between Shepperton and Walton. It was an idyllic setting with a lake lapping the back garden boundary. A residence association was formed. I was elected treasurer and each of the 15 houses contributed the princely sum of £1 membership fee. Church-wise, we joined a group of Christians from Woking Baptist Church and reopened a small Anglican church building in Upper Halliford.

It became clear to me that Botley's Park Hospital required urgent attention. In contrast to Ely Hospital with its old buildings, Botley's Park was located in beautiful parkland, with the original mansion as the core and patients housed in relatively modern units dotted around the estate with day accommodation on the ground floor and beds on the first floor. My concern mounted when, on being taken on a tour of the hospital by the head of nursing who had not long been in post, I witnessed a remarkable scene – a patient wearing only a toy helmet hosing another patient with a fire hydrant while the charge nurse of the unit was a passive onlooker! The problems became even more obvious when a young female consultant was appointed and became totally frustrated at the lack of co-operation from the medical superintendent in developing rehabilitation programmes – some of the children never left their beds. In the light of the Ely Report, I found that the deficiencies highlighted in that report were more applicable to Botley's Park than Ely Hospital. Clearly Botley's Park had very serious problems with dysfunctional leadership. The hospital secretary, who was of retiring age, took my advice and retired. His replacement was an exceptionally able and mature administrator who had returned from the Bahamas and was seeking re-entry to the NHS. An independent inquiry, set up by the Regional Hospital Board and chaired by a barrister, instigated fundamental changes in senior management affecting nursing and medical services at Botley's Park. The head of nursing was transferred to a staff post elsewhere in the region, the medical superintendent relinquished his leadership role, reverting to being a consultant, with the new young consultant becoming chairman of the medical committee for Botley's Park. The inquiry sat for five days during which I lost nearly a stone in weight! Improvements in care followed. Children who had never left their beds were being taught and responded by learning simple skills for the first time. I recall the heart-warming spectacle of young patients rendering a simple hymn tune with hand bells at the annual service for patients and relatives held in the main hall at Botley's Park – a truly uplifting experience. I gave the sermon on that occasion – the story of Zacheus climbing the tree to get a better view of Jesus. The chairman of the HMC complimented me afterwards with the comment "you would have made a good bishop, Evans"!

These mental institutions were, by and large, closed and isolated communities so I was thrilled when approached by a film director and friend living in the Guildford area with a proposal to raise funds for a small hall to be built at Botley's Park as a communal facility. I readily agreed to match their fund-raising efforts by committing NHS resources to implementing the scheme. The launch was a gala dinner held in the main hall at Botley's Park – the catering provided by the hospital staff. Circular tables, seating twelve to fifteen guests, were 'purchased' by wealthy donors. Entertainment was provided voluntarily by an opera singer from Covent Garden. The event could have been a disaster – Fanny Cradock with her husband Johnnie, of TV cookery fame, arrived with her guests but walked out when the first course of a simple salad was served. The *Daily Mirror* reported the incident, and the money rolled in! I was also approached by the owner of a market garden purchased from Botley's Park under a government policy to dispose of farms and gardens in the NHS with a proposal to develop a golf course which could only be built with additional land leased from the hospital. Unfortunately the regional hospital board did not share my enthusiasm for the scheme!

Another problem area related to Woking Hospital which had suffered in status following the development of St Peters Hospital and the opening of a new maternity unit there and the closure of maternity beds at Woking. In contrast to the strong local involvement of the public in other small hospitals in the group, Woking Hospital was bereft of voluntary participation such as a League of Friends. This deficiency was remedied when the Woking Conservative Club agreed to form a League of Friends for Woking Hospital with the caveat that, at times of an election, their priorities would be political rather than support for the hospital! These arrangements worked well for both parties.

On another memorable occasion, a member of the HMC burst into my office waving a copy of the local newspaper with a blazing front page headline 'Husband thrown out of labour ward'. The husband had wanted to be present at the birth of his first child but had been physically ejected by the consultant obstetrician who was nearing retirement age – it was not common practice and official policy for fathers to be present in those days. I conveyed sincere apologies to the aggrieved father with the added advice, "Next time, you may wish to have your child born in Kingston-upon-Thames where a more enlightened policy already prevails".

Another problem area related to Holloway Sanatorium located in Virginia Waters. It was an interesting building – a Grade I listed Gothic-inspired Victorian ex-asylum and a veritable death trap in the event of a fire. Before the NHS it provided psychiatric care for the wealthy and privileged. It even had its own railway siding. One painful experience remains in my memory to this day. A senior nurse was retiring after years of service at Holloway during which he occupied a hospital house, but the local authority would not grant him a council house unless he and his family were rendered homeless. So the HMC and I were party to the unedifying spectacle of sending the bailiffs in to repossess the hospital house in the full glare of adverse publicity. The HMC, because of the high cost of housing in this area, could not recruit key staff without providing a hospital house. It was a very distressing experience not least because, within a year or so, the regional hospital board declared their intention to close the hospital. Furthermore, the whole matter could have been resolved amicably with a more co-operative attitude by the local housing authority.

Another aspect of my time in north-west Surrey involved preparation and advice on the forthcoming major reorganisation of the NHS in 1974 – the most fundamental change since 1948. The proposals in England merged the tripartite division of the NHS into one structure with two tiers below the Department of Health – Regional Health Boards and Area Health Authorities (the latter supported by executive district teams where appropriate). Family practitioner committees replaced executive councils: GPs, chemists and opticians, and local government health services: medical officers of public health, district nursing, ambulance services and school health services were transferred to the new Area Health Authorities. In Wales, the Welsh Regional Hospital Board was dissolved, with Area Health Authorities undertaking some of the responsibilities exercised by RHBs in England being directly accountable to the Welsh Office. The emergence of the Welsh Assembly with devolved responsibilities for health was to come later. Joint Liaison Committees (JLCs) were established at chief officer level to advise on the structure of the new authorities including sensitive issues such as boundaries and catchment areas and which of the proposed AHAs would have district teams as, for example, in Surrey. I was the chairman of a JLC but was increasingly frustrated by the lack of progress in reaching agreement on vital issues – everyone was arguing his own case with self interest in mind. At a particular meeting of the JLC, with time running out, I declared with exasperation from the chair: "Gentlemen, this is not good enough. It is a *cabolach*." There was a stunned silence, while I explained that the word in Welsh meant a mess, and a very big mess as only the Welsh can create at times! Everyone came to their senses and our agreed recommendations with some reservations were accepted and implemented.

During the three years in north-west Surrey, I continued to enjoy participating in courses organised by the King's Fund International Hospital Federation for overseas administrators, giving talks at national, regional and local conferences regarding the implications of the forthcoming reorganisation for existing authorities, local government, especially Social Services, and voluntary bodies. Also, on more specific themes such as 'Strategic Planning for Health Services' at the University of Manchester and 'Introducing Change' to the Industrial Society public services group. I was a member of the DHSS steering group on a NHS reorganisation film, as well as having further papers published in professional journals.

Under the 1974 reorganisation, all existing chief officers had to apply for designated posts in the new structure – a rather unsettling experience for individuals and their families, and part of the human cost, underestimated in my opinion, involved in every major reorganisation. Multidisciplinary courses were arranged for existing chief officers and I benefited immensely from such a course at the University of York, not least from the contribution made by medical officers of health and chief ambulance officers. The course had the privilege of hearing from the vice chancellor on the development of the

University of York who, in answer to the question how was he able to reconcile educational concepts with architectural design replied that he had never worked so hard in all his life but had been blessed with architects not preoccupied with an esoteric monument but a building reflecting educational concepts for future uses. The vice chancellor had to define the purpose of every room and space in the building and the result is a truly beautiful university campus. His observations reminded me of a comment by a consultant physician at West Middlesex Hospital: "you administrators have to live with your mistakes. We bury ours." Some modern hospitals in the UK have had to bear heavy costs because of poor design and construction deficiencies.

I could have happily remained in Surrey and the only post I applied for in the reorganised structure was that of chief administrator and secretary to the board of the South Glamorgan Health Authority (Teaching). I was appointed and returned to Cardiff in September 1973 having achieved the ambition to be a chief administrator in the reorganised NHS.

12

The top of the ladder in
South Glamorgan (1973–83)

I FELT ELATED when I was appointed to the South Glamorgan
Area Health Authority – a teaching, single district AHA with
some of the responsibilities of RHBs in England, and directly
accountable to the Welsh Office. The AHA was responsible
for providing comprehensive healthcare to nearly 400,000
people in South Glamorgan and a wide range of regional and
sub-regional services for up to 1.5 million in the Principality.
During the latter half of 1973 the AHA operated in shadow
form, taking over full responsibility on 1 April 1974 – a period
taken up appointing various statutory committees such as
the family practitioner committee, which replaced executive
councils, and chief officers and senior staff. A special service
to mark the handing over of healthcare to the new authority
was held in the chapel of the University Hospital of Wales on
Sunday, 31 March 1974, during which the congregation stood
and declared:

> We have assembled together in the presence of Almighty God, to
> offer to him, through our Lord Jesus Christ, our worship, praise,
> and thanksgiving; and in particular to give thanks to him for
> all that has been achieved by the National Health Service since
> its inception in 1948. And we give thanks also for all who seek
> to bring healing and wholeness to the sick and suffering. We
> commend to Almighty God the work that is being done at present
> and will be done in the future in the new structure of the Health
> Service, asking his blessing on all who serve to promote it.

The chairman of the AHA was Raymond Cory, a fine gentleman with business interests in shipping and Cardiff Docks who had previously been a member of the board of governors of united Cardiff hospitals. The vice-chairman for an initial period of four years was Principal Arnold James who had served on the Cardiff HMC, Cardiff & District HMC and the University of Wales (Cardiff) HMC. The authority's modus operandi embraced an open style of management and only in exceptional circumstances, such as disciplinary matters, would the media be excluded from its deliberations. A dialogue with the media on health service matters was encouraged. With the emphasis on team building, there were times of tension between myself and the other six chief officers who were accountable to the chairman: medical, nursing, finance, dental, pharmaceutical and works, over which I had co-ordinating responsibilities – the designation of chief executive officer was only introduced in the NHS later. Having enjoyed CEO status for three years in north-west Surrey, I felt at times I was managing with one arm tied behind my back but freely admitted to being a benign dictator, but always open to discussion, and fully accountable to peer review and higher authority.

Although familiar with the Cardiff scene I had underestimated the problems inherited by the AHA. On the plus side, the UHW had been opened by Her Majesty the Queen in November 1971 – a Rolls Royce which only highlighted deficiencies in other hospitals especially Cardiff Royal Infirmary. Originally, the CRI was to close when the UHW opened but, following government policy to expand medical education in the UK, the medical student intake in Cardiff was doubled from 75 to 150 per annum, and the CRI was kept open. A fire had emptied the CRI's maternity unit in Glossop Terrace but, after costly renovations, it remained unoccupied for a long period because of difficulty in recruiting midwives thereby putting maternity beds at UHW and St David's Hospital under considerable pressure. From the outset the

AHA faced enormous pressures to rationalize its services and reduce costs – the other AHAs in Wales claiming that South Glamorgan had received more than its fair share of capital and revenue money. It was a difficult wicket to bat on in the full glare of media coverage. We felt we were in a goldfish bowl with the public and media rightly giving high priority to health care issues. In contrast South Glamorgan, as a teaching AHA, was committed to the pursuit of standards of excellence in relation to patient care, education and training, and research. The early years were tough but standards were improved in the longer-stay units providing geriatric, psychiatric and mental handicap care. Priority was given to developing community health services and health education; an improved ambulance service with a new control centre and the latest technology was opened in Tŷ Bronna, an ex-nurses home, at Glan Ely Hospital. Lower costs and improved efficiency were achieved in the three major acute hospitals: UHW, CRI and Llandough, by shedding some 300 posts so that no more than 75 per cent of revenue expenditure was devoted to manpower and that all new developments were fully funded. The CRI west wing was reopened for acute and rehabilitation geriatric care, and to accommodate the STI clinic hitherto located in appalling accommodation. With the director of Social Services for the county of South Glamorgan, I made it clear from the outset that health and social services staff were expected to co-operate fully at all levels and joint mechanisms were set up for planning and operational purposes.

However, the authority was not successful in achieving major improvements by closing some units and providing alternative provision in other existing under-used units. There was overwhelming opposition, during the periods of public consultation, by the public, staff and unions to such proposals affecting Barry, Lansdowne, Glan Ely, St David's and Prince of Wales, Rhydlafar. I recall meeting George Thomas MP, who bewailed the fact that the AHA was concentrating the closures in his constituency at Glan Ely, Lansdowne and St

David's. I made the preposterous suggestion that perhaps we should move the Casualty Department from CRI to St David's Hospital. The MP's reply, a classic party political stance, was "Better not, that's Prime Minister territory"! I later related that encounter to the Prime Minister and Mrs Callaghan when they came to a prize-giving ceremony at the UHW. The PM chuckled and added, "Yes, that would be George".

The AHA's long-term strategic goal was to concentrate acute services in two major complexes, at UHW and Llandough, supported by peripheral community or specialist hospitals, and by 2010 this has now been largely achieved. There are now new hospitals at Barry, and St David's and the following units, inherited by the AHA in 1974, have been closed and their sites disposed of and redeveloped mainly for housing: Barry Community, Barry Neale Kent, Barry Amy Evans, Children's ENT, Sully, St Mary's, Lord Pontypridd, Prince of Wales, Rhydlafar; Royal Hamadryad and Wm Nicholls Home. The CRI has remained empty for years but proposals have now been made for this valuable site to be redeveloped when funds are available for primary care, community care, and outpatient clinics to relieve pressure on UHW to serve the east area of Cardiff. The Cardiff & Vale University Health Board has recently announced the closure of Rookwood Hospital – the only spinal rehabilitation unit in Wales – and the work there to be absorbed into existing units, probably Llandough Hospital. The current philosophy is to keep the patient out of hospital where possible or for the minimum period in hospital. Prevention and health education have gained momentum – who would have believed years ago that a ban on smoking in public places could be achieved by legislation. Much more remains to be done in respect of lifestyles with increasing problems of obesity, alcohol and drug-related infirmities. In the meantime the boundaries of medical science are extended apace with inevitable increasing demands on scarce resources. Strategic decisions are going to be made regarding the provision of special centres of excellence, e.g. reducing the centres for paediatric cardiothoracic surgery. The care of the elderly will add particular pressures on health and social services resources.

There are many memorable events I recall during my period with South Glamorgan AHA.

Firstly the visit by Princess Margaret to Velindre Hospital to open a new ward appropriately named the Princess Margaret Suite.

Also my appearance at the House of Commons' Select Committee on complaints investigated by the ombudsman. It related to a complaint involving the University Hospital of Wales (Cardiff) HMC regarding a patient who had been admitted three times for cardiac surgery but, for various reasons, the operation had been cancelled on each occasion. The first question was addressed to Mr Cory the AHA chairman who explained that he was newly appointed and that the chairman of the HMC had retired. Dr Skone (AMO) and Mary Worster (ANO) replied in similar veins. I was able to say that my equivalent predecessor, Mr Norman Popplewell, was in Australia. Having been assured that every case of a cancelled operation was fully investigated, the Select Committee discharged us with the comment, "we've got the wrong people before us"! A daunting experience.

I also recollect a press conference at UHW when Mervyn 'the swerve' Davies, one of the all time great No. 8 rugby internationals, was discharged from the UHW, after collapsing with a brain haemorrhage during a Cup final at Cardiff Arms Park. In contrast to my experience ten years earlier when Ted Dexter was admitted to West Middlesex Hospital, the media now co-operated fully by responding to daily bulletins regarding his progress. Mervyn Davies, in a wheelchair, was accompanied by a consultant neurosurgeon and the ward sister. I expressed the heartfelt good wishes of all that Mervyn Davies was now well enough to be discharged, and thanked the media and the patient for their co-operation.

Another memorable moment came on the day that Peter Grey, the area works officer, reported that a large chunk of masonry had fallen off the main structure of UHW. Extensive tests subsequently showed that areas of mosaic cladding and supporting concrete beams were corroded – a design and construction failure which cost the AHA £6½ million to correct with money diverted from patient care. At a hastily convened press conference, the BBC's Vincent Kane, with the cameras rolling, opened with the question "Can you be sure Mr Evans that the UHW is safe?" Involvement with the media demanded a lot of time and effort on my part but I considered it an important facet of my responsibilities and all the income I received for my many appearances on TV or radio was donated to the Medical Research Fund.

The 1979 winter of discontent was a particularly difficult period with trade unions taking strike action and using patients as pawns in a power struggle with the government. At times the unions' demands were extreme. Staff were expected to be paid for doing nothing and sometimes their action would be stage managed with the connivance of the media to gain maximum publicity.

I gained immense satisfaction from developing the talents of individual officers, some of these went on to achieve chief officer status – the area ambulance officer became a regional chief in England, and two of my deputies in South Glamorgan became chief administrators in Wales. I believed that *the* most important single task among my wide ranging responsibilities was the appointment of staff. I failed with respect to one senior administrative appointment, and it cost me dearly in terms of heartache.

In the wider context, I continued to give talks at various conferences and at the King's Fund Centre and had papers on health-related topics published. I was a member of the Trethowan Committee's report on the role of psychologists in the health services in 1977. I was one of the UK representatives at two international seminars in 1975 and 1977, sponsored by the Kellogs Foundation and the King's Fund, to study healthcare systems in the USA, Canada, Australia, New Zealand and the UK. Despite widely differing methods of providing and funding health care, the underlying problems were similar – escalating costs and inadequate funding. These seminars confirmed in my mind that the *comprehensive* healthcare provision through the NHS with state funding and involving the private sector gave the best overall value for money – a view amply confirmed in later life as a major consumer of the NHS. I also had the privilege of being the chief administrator's representative on the policy committee of the Association of Health Authorities in England and Wales. By the early 1980s it was acknowledged that a major review of the management arrangements set up under the 1974 reorganisation of the NHS was called for, with greater emphasis on placing the patient first. I was seconded to the Welsh Office for three months to advise the Secretary of State for Wales. This was another enriching experience.

Despite all the pressures, I really loved the job – its challenges and variety. Above all, it was to do with people. I was a natural workaholic with high standards and demanded the same commitment from others. But calamity struck in September 1979, when I broke down while having an informal discussion with the chairman in his office at the Temple of Peace. Sufferers of severe clinical depression will know that episodes can recur with varying intensity and length but, with the help of modern drugs and medical expertise, there is light at the end of the tunnel. Eventually blue skies return, sometimes after weeks and months of distress during which progress is varied, and one feels as though one step forward is followed by two steps back. By 1982, after another severe episode of depression triggered by influenza – by now I was on lithium which caused kidney damage and left me with an additional health problem of diabetic insipidus, excessive thirst – I felt enough was enough. I was also conscious of the history of depression on my mother's side of the family.

On 2 June 1983 I wrote to the chairman of the Authority seeking early retirement on medical grounds. It was not a difficult decision – just an end to another chapter in my life.

TEL. 761250.

15 HEOL ST. DENYS,
LISVANE,
CARDIFF,
CF4 5RU

2nd June 1983

Dear Raymond,

Further to our informal discussions since I commenced sick leave on 16th March last, I wish to apply for early retirement on medical grounds with effect from 30th September 1983. My doctor has provided the necessary report for the Medical Adviser, DHSS Superannuation Branch.

Naturally, I have mixed feelings at this time bearing in mind I have spent nearly 33 happy and demanding years in the National Health Service – the last 9½ years as Chief Administrator and Secretary to the South Glamorgan Health Authority under your chairmanship.

However, I am certain it is the right decision both from my own and the Authority's viewpoints.

yours sincerely

Adrian
(ADRIAN M. EVANS)

Raymond Cory Esq. CBE.
Chairman,
South Glamorgan Health Authority.

PART THREE

RETIREMENT

13

Life after early retirement on medical grounds

LEAVING ASIDE EPISODES of ill-health, I have spent the last 28 years living life to the full, being involved in Christian voluntary work and participating in non-Christian activities. Until 2009 I enjoyed gardening but those physical demands have now been out-sourced. I served for a period on the national steering group of the European Commission's network of district projects on disability – an interesting experience because it highlighted the potential and real contribution of the disabled to society if given the opportunity to do so. I was invited by the professor of education at Cardiff University to be a part-time tutor in 1983/4 on a masters' degree course. That was a rewarding experience, not least an encounter with a particular student from northern Nigeria, a devout Muslim, who suddenly disappeared following a coup in that country. I became increasingly uneasy regarding his dissertation which took the form of an application to the EU Commission in Brussels for significant funds to up-grade his school.

I maintained my interest in missionary activities, particularly with the Overseas Missionary Fellowship (OMF) – an international multi-denominational missionary society serving south-east Asia, previously known as the China Inland Mission (CIM) before their expulsion from mainland China by the communist government in 1951. In addition to serving on the OMF's south-west regional council, I was for a period the chairman of the Cornford House management committee – a residential home in Kent providing nursing care for elderly retired OMF missionaries. This latter commitment was a particularly rewarding and humbling experience. I met warriors who had faced incredible hardships, including some who had been interned during the Japanese occupation of China in the Second World War. My NHS experience was relevant because Cornford House required dual approval by the local health authority and social services – it passed with flying colours. These responsibilities entailed a three- to four-day visit to Kent every quarter which included briefing the OMF's headquarters in Sevenoaks, a meeting of the management committee, interaction with the residents and staff over meals, and a personal chat with each resident. On one occasion, a resident in her nineties responded to my knock on her bedroom door, and the following dialogue ensued:

Resident: Where did you work in China?

A: I've never had the opportunity to visit China. (I felt demoted immediately!)

Resident: Where did you work in south-east Asia?

A: I've never had the opportunity to serve in south-east Asia. (A further demotion)

Resident: When did you become a member of OMF?

A: I've never sought that privilege but have been an active supporter. (Further demotion)

Resident: What are you doing here and who are you?

A: (Now feeling totally demoted) I'm just helping to run Cornford House and I've come to see if you are alright.

I visited Cornford House soon after the October 1987 hurricane which uprooted six of the seven oaks in Sevenoaks and surrounding pine trees which were mown down like matchsticks. Cornford House was spared damage but one resident gave a graphic description of how, in the midst of the storm, she lay in bed while the flat roof over her bedroom kept moving but never took off, in answer to fervent prayer.

During the past 27 years, I have served as an elder at three independent evangelical churches in Cardiff – at Heath Evangelical Church, at Highfields Church (I was a founding elder in 1986) and at Thornhill Community Church and Centre for a period of some six years, retiring as their first elder emeritus in 2001. Edwina and I returned to Highfields Church as members in November 2008. The church had been greatly blessed while we had been at Thornhill, and has retained its core biblical values as a mission-centred fellowship.

In terms of leisure activity, Edwina and I took up golf but we were never very good at it. We enjoyed the exercise but mutually agreed that golf was a great sport but not to be taken seriously unless one was feeling very competitive and good at it! In the early years of my retirement, Huw was a keen fisherman and a member of the Welsh disabled team. We spent many a happy, if frustrating, holidays in Ireland and Scotland trying to land the elusive salmon, but without success. We have enjoyed holidays in the USA, Canada, Australia and Europe, but in the last few years have not travelled beyond Portugal because of health-related problems and the cost of insurance cover.

One particular incident occurred while on holiday in the Algarve which I count as the most embarrassing incident in my whole life – the antidote to such an event is humour, although there was nothing funny about it at the time. At about 1.30 a.m. in our apartment on the 5th floor of Hotel Portobelo, Vilamoura I trotted off to the loo and, in a half sleep, opened the wrong door and found myself locked out in the corridor – dressed only in pyjama shorts, and without my glasses and hearing aids, which were on the bedside table, and teeth, which were in the bathroom, and dishevelled hair – I was not a pretty sight. I rang the bell and thumped the door to the apartment without any response from Edwina sleeping blissfully in the bedroom. After an hour or so I crept downstairs to the hotel's reception area, explained my predicament to the night porter and requested a spare key. A further embarrassment occurred when the night porter asked me for the number of my apartment but I could not remember it! The porter checked the records, called the maintenance man on duty, who escorted me back to the apartment at around 3 a.m. In creeping back into bed, Edwina woke and listening to my tale of woe, dismissed it as a dream, to which I replied, "it's no dream – it's reality". The footnote to that saga was that we had a great holiday, and lived happily ever after!

Health-wise, Edwina and I have, in keeping with the ageing process, made increasing demands on the NHS. We and our son Huw are registered with a first-class group practice with GPs who are sensitive and sympathetic to individual needs and well organised – the family have never failed to obtain an urgent appointment within 24 hours. I continue to experience episodes of clinical depression. In 2005 I was admitted to the UHW having collapsed at home due to a severe depressive episode. I was seen by a psychiatrist, given a change of drugs and within weeks was a new man, even feeling I could manage the NHS again! On another occasion, I was admitted as an emergency, having collapsed in one of Huw's student houses after struggling to replace a lavatory seat. Initially, they thought it was a heart attack but it turned out to be a massive cramp of the chest muscles. A few days stay in the thoracic/heart ward brought home to me the incredible advances made in that field of medicine. Some five years ago I was admitted to the UHW for a removal of a lump on the side of my neck. The growth proved benign but the experience underlined the enormous pressures on the acute in-patient services in the NHS. I had to ring the ward to check if a bed was available on the day of my admission. I was second on the operations' list for the following day but the first case took eight hours and I was discharged home and re-admitted a week later – again having to check if a bed was available.

It was a very busy ward shared by ENT and oral surgery but two of the beds in my nine-bed ward were blocked by patients awaiting alternative non-acute care. Another aspect was the detailed explanation given to me on the risks involved – the dire consequences if some of the nerve ends surrounding the tumour were severed. No doubt this was to avoid any claim by the patient or relatives if anything went wrong but, in my view, it underlined the urgency of establishing a non-adversarial mechanism for dealing with litigation when errors do occur in medical care. While an in-patient, I had the opportunity of reading my hospital case notes, some five inches thick – very interesting and revealing!

I was first diagnosed with prostate cancer in December 2002. It had spread beyond the prostate so surgery was not an option, but it responded to hormone and radiotherapy treatment. In March 2008 the cancer became active again and scans in August 2009 revealed it had spread to the spine and later to the pelvis. It failed to respond to additional hormone treatment or to a clinical trial of a new drug. Hence from June to October 2010, the chemotherapy treatment docetaxel began – the same treatment that the Lockerbie bomber Al-Megrahi received in Tripoli. My two first cousins, the sons of my uncle, Rev. D J Williams, were also diagnosed and successfully treated with prostate cancer in 2010 and we are all participating in the UK Genetic Prostate Cancer Study by the Institute of Cancer Research in London.

Bearing in mind that so much information regarding healthcare is now available in the public domain, including the latest breakthroughs in treatments, the attitudes of healthcare staff towards patients have been transformed. Information regarding my treatment has been excellent and the onus is now on the patient and/or relatives to seek further information if they wish.

The pressures on NHS resources are inevitably going to increase and the cutting out of waste is a top priority with patients playing their part too. A recent publication,

'Community Pharmacy Wales', highlighted the scandal of the £50 million lost each year in medicine wastage. A renewed emphasis on prevention is called for, coupled with a concerted attack on the disparities which increasingly exist within the NHS – both in terms of standards of care and variation in costs incurred. A recent report from the National Audit Office highlighted the failure of the NHS to spend its cancer budget wisely 'with some parts of the country spending three times as much as others on each patient, with most of the difference unexplained and little evidence that treatment is any better'. There is also evidence of a deterioration in basic care for the elderly within the NHS.

I have serious reservations about the latest proposals for the reorganisation of the NHS in England, particularly giving GP consortiums significant budgetary control. The commissioning of health care services is a multi-disciplinary exercise involving relevant expertise – general practice, hospital specialists, university medical schools, community medicine, public health, healthcare economists, consumer representatives, together with nursing, financial and administrative expertise in healthcare management. The proposed NHS commissioning board will need some form of mechanism at regional and local level for interacting with local health boards and other providers. Furthermore, the commissioning consortiums should not only be involved in purchasing services but be involved in the implementation of healthcare developments, both capital and revenue, and the monitoring of healthcare provisions, especially deficiencies, at local level. The interaction of the commissioning consortiums with local health boards and other providers should be subject to public and media scrutiny.

Even if these radical and controversial measures prove successful and that there are commensurate financial savings and improvements in efficiency in Wales, Scotland and Northern Ireland, the NHS faces a daunting future. The pressures for financing the needs of the NHS will be so much greater in future as new and improved aspects of healthcare are identified and introduced, coupled with an ongoing commitment to improving existing services to a satisfactory level throughout the UK. The NHS is meant to be a national comprehensive healthcare service, yet there are increasing disparities in provision within the UK. Perhaps we have yet, as a nation, to have a full debate about what we can and cannot afford in healthcare.

It has been calculated that the NHS requires 'about four per cent more money every year to keep pace with rising demand, new technologies and an ageing population'. Even allowing for savings and more efficient ways of working, a fundamental review of the basis for funding the NHS is urgent as the gap between need and available finance widens increasingly in future years.

*

3 May 2011

The last few months have been a testing time. The chemotherapy arrested the prostate cancer – the PSA fell from 200 to 40 – but had the effect of undermining the efficacy of the drugs I was taking for clinical depression. I suffered a serious relapse in December 2010 – depression is so corrosive on the mind, body and soul. On being seen by two psychiatrists as an urgent case, having collapsed at home and just wanted to die, they arranged for me to attend the day hospital for one day every week to monitor progress. After 11 weeks I was discharged with the new medication having worked wonders and the depression completely gone. Furthermore, if I suffered a further relapse I was to attend the Hafan Day Hospital without delay. Since May 2007, I have been participating in mood disorders research conducted by the bipolar disorder research network team at Cardiff University and the University of Birmingham.

In relation to the prostate cancer, the PSA (a crude indication of cancer activity) had increased to 130 by early February this year but decreased to 112 by mid April. A change of steroid has been very beneficial to the extent that, at the outpatient clinic on 20 April, I asked the consultant oncologist if I could go on a fortnight's holiday to the Algarve at the end of May (the GP was in favour subject to the oncologist's advice) and, whether I should dispense the fortnight timeshare holidays in October. The oncologist's reply was brilliant, 'Be optimistic about holidays but pessimistic regarding financial matters'! Never ask a doctor how long one is likely to live – the Lord has that in hand.

But there will come a day, sooner or later, when my earthly journey will end. My faith and trust in the Lord is unshakeable and I have no fear of death – I look forward to a glorious eternal fellowship with the Lord – free from the blemishes of this earthly life in a fallen world. Thanks be to God – diolch iddo.

30 August 2011 – Life in a wheelchair
My life took an unexpected turn on Saturday, 23 July 2011 when my legs could not support my weight. I was admitted as an emergency to Llandough Hospital, Cardiff, transferred the following day to the UHW, Cardiff for an MRI scan and, later that evening, to Velindre Hospital where I remained an in-patient until discharged home on 10 August 2011.

The initial diagnosis of partial paralysis in both legs due to pressure on the spinal cord caused by prostate cancer was changed following a review by oncologists, radiologists and orthopaedic specialists of the MRI scans taken some 15 months ago and on 24 July 2011. It was agreed that degeneration of the lower spine was causing the partial paralysis. Furthermore, surgery was not an option, to my relief, nor radiotherapy other than a dose given to relieve pain.

The physiotherapists taught me how to get in and out of bed to a wheelchair and how to exercise my legs and lower abdomen muscles. The occupational therapist visited our home and discussed with Edwina the requirements for my discharge – converting the dining room on the ground floor into a bedroom. The social worker from Cardiff City Council, but based in the hospital, arranged the care package for my needs at home.

On discharge, I wrote to the chief executive of the Velindre NHS Trust, the ward manager, medical, nursing, physiotherapy, occupational therapy, social worker, ward clerk, voluntary worker, and the discharge co-ordinator, in the following terms:

> I am full of praise and gratitude for the care and treatment received while an in-patient here. All the staff, without exception, have been friendly, kind, sensitive, encouraging and professional – despite times of great pressure. The food has been excellent – I feel I'm staying in the best hotel in Cardiff! The 14-day menu has provided a variety of choice at breakfast, lunch and supper, all prepared in the ward kitchen and hot and delicious when served. The emphasis on ward cleaning is another feature which I've observed – I've been tested twice for MRSA! The communication with patients by various professional groups: medical, nursing, physiotherapy, occupational therapy and social worker has been excellent, and the communication between professional staff, expressed in teamwork, is exceptionally good. The teamwork also extends beyond the hospital setting, e.g. the case conference to plan my discharge, with my wife and son Huw (who is in a wheelchair) present, included a district nurse from our GP practice in Whitchurch Road, Cardiff. The provisions for discharge could not be better. The care package included carers and equipment: an adjustable bed with air mattress, hoist and mini ramps for home. Social Services cannot provide a 'STEDY' for community care, and we have purchased one ourselves – it is the one bit of equipment that has helped me most since my admission with partial paralysis of both legs. I have spent my professional life in the NHS and was Chief Administrator of South Glamorgan Health Authority from 1973–83. It has been a real tonic to have received such excellent care and treatment here. Part of the tonic was the coffee and cakes morning arranged by the physiotherapists in the ward on the ground floor and visiting the gem of a garden developed by Carol and her friend

George, both voluntary workers. Thank you all so much for everything. I shall continue to be looked after as an outpatient, now on palliative care for prostate cancer.

I was seen by my consultant oncologist, Dr John Staffurth, as an outpatient on 25 August. Although my PSA had risen to 230, I was reassured to learn that, comparing the recent bone scan with one taken 18 months ago, the prostate cancer had not spread at an alarming rate. My progress will be reviewed in two months but with immediate recall if symptoms deteriorate. Arrangements are in hand for me to receive on-going help from a community-based physiotherapist.

Finally, I feel that this is an appropriate time to end my jottings of *A Life's Journey*. I now value each day knowing that in God's time, I will be called Home '…into an inheritance that can never perish, spoil or fade – kept in heaven… '(1 Peter 1 v.4). During my recent in-patient stay, I studied the Psalms and the following simple yet profound verse engulfed my mind, body and soul: 'I lie down and sleep; I wake again, because the Lord sustains me.' (Psalm 3 v.5) That verse says it all. Amen.

27 April 2012

I was admitted as an emergency to the University Hospital of Wales on 31 January, my legs having given way. An MRI scan confirmed the problem was due to degeneration of the lower spine – which had necessitated my admission to hospital in August last year. I was discharged on 3 February and referred by the Macmillan nurse at UHW to the Palliative Care Team of the George Thomas Hospice Care.

Meanwhile, I have been delighted to learn that research into the family background on my mother's side by my brother Trefor has discovered family member Jedediah Richards (1784–1838), who was 'A famous hymn writer, educationalist and peripatetic philosopher' according to information in the *Bywgraffiadur Cymreig* published in 1940 by Cymdeithas y

Cymmrodorion. My cousin Ieuan, only son of D J Davies, has also found out that ancestor Timothy Richards (1845–1919) wrote a book called *Forty-five years in China: Reminiscences* and it is available on the Amazon website. His was a remarkable story with a graphic account and insight into the state of China and its struggles to improve during that period.

Finally, Joe, our eldest grandson, aged 21, now living in Bristol recently passed his driving test and spends two days a week here helping three disabled relatives – his grandparents and Uncle Huw! God's provision.

14

Palliative medicine and end of life care

THE PROSTATE CANCER Cardiff support group asked me to write about end of life care – a sensitive but all-important matter for we all must face death at some time or other. Surely, our desire would be that we die with dignity and with compassion shown by those who care for us. Martin Luther said "We should familiarise ourselves with death during our lifetime...", a view endorsed by Billy Graham in his book, *Nearing Home: Life, Faith, and Finishing Well.*

I was referred to the George Thomas Hospice Care on 3 February 2012 by a Macmillan nurse after my discharge from the University Hospital of Wales. I have been, since February 2012, under the care of the Palliative Care Team (PCT) of the George Thomas Hospice Care – a service complementary to the excellent care provided by the GP and specialist teams in oncology, psychiatry and ENT at Velindre Hospital, Hafan Day Unit at Whitchurch Hospital, and the ENT department at University Hospital of Wales respectively.

The impact of the PCT has been significant. My prostate cancer was first diagnosed 10 years ago, but, at 80 years of age, I look remarkably well and have a current PSA of 2,200! I am enjoying a quality of life that I did not anticipate was possible a year or so ago. The PCT service is on call at all times which is a big relief and reassurance to the family.

This is my first experience of being looked after by healthcare staff who are specialists in palliative care for patients such as myself with incurable conditions needing end of life care, and it has been a revelation. The Royal College of Physicians established palliative care as a distinct medical speciality in 1987 and we are fortunate to have in Cardiff an international authority, namely Baroness Finlay of Llandaff.

The initial visit was devoted to explaining how the team worked and giving information on the extensive range of experts and activities at their headquarters, within the grounds of Whitchurch Hospital, Tŷ George Thomas, available to patients and relatives. George Thomas Hospice Care has specialists in healthcare, social work, welfare rights, bereavement and counselling for adults and children and a range of activities in Tŷ George Thomas: a breathlessness management group, multi-disciplinary day centre, bereavement group, outpatients clinic, complementary therapies, social interactions, mutual support and friendship and respite for carers.

I had to agree formally for the team to have access to my NHS medical records and to have permission to liaise direct with the GP and hospital specialists and Social Services as the need arose.

The first visit by Dr Margred Capel, consultant in palliative medicine, was most illuminating and instructive. It included a thorough medical examination and assessment of my disabilities but also ranged over aspects of care, e.g. taking exercise but resting after lunch even if I didn't feel tired, listening to my body, pacing all activities – all challenging to my normal attitude to life! Currently I get around the house with walking aids, but activities such as attending church on a Sunday morning, a midweek men's fellowship on Wednesday morning, the occasional Probus meeting on a Thursday morning with lunch, and the odd shopping in town are in a wheelchair.

Karen Smith, clinical nurse specialist, visits every fortnight or so. We both look forward to her arrival – she is a tonic. My progress is reviewed in general and in relation to specific health indicators, e.g. fatigue, pain, diet, etc. Edwina is often more objective and accurate in responding to these issues.

Other members of the palliative care team have made significant contribution to my care and well-being – the physiotherapists regarding physical exercises to strengthen the legs, thigh and stomach muscles and the occupational therapists providing aids for the home, e.g. ramps, support aids and timely advice on the purchase and installation of a chair lift. Edwina and I are so grateful for all their contributions.

We particularly value the sensitive and dignified way they respect our expectations regarding care during this final phase of our lives. We are committed Christians who enjoy fellowship in a vibrant church, Highfields, and support from family, neighbours and friends. In contrast, the Secretary of State for Health, Jeremy Hunt, recently announced a scheme to identify loneliness black spots across the country, as it is one of the fastest growing health problems. The mapping project will enable health services, councils and other agencies to come to the aid of elderly people in areas where they suffer most acutely from isolation. The number of elderly people who suffer loneliness is growing rapidly partly a result of the ageing population and partly because children are moving further away from their family homes. Research showed more than half of those over the age of 75 live alone, with one in ten saying they feel intensely lonely.

The George Thomas Hospice Care is a registered charity dependent on the contributions of individuals and agencies to maintain their invaluable services, with an army of volunteers in their charity shops etc. supporting the hospice staff.

The demand for their services will inevitably increase as patients such as me will be cared for in the community rather than hospital or a care home and this at a time when the NHS is facing enormous financial problems with competing claims for its limited resources.

Finally, all the income accruing to myself from the publication of this book will be donated equally to the two charities, George Thomas Hospice Care and Cancer Research Wales.

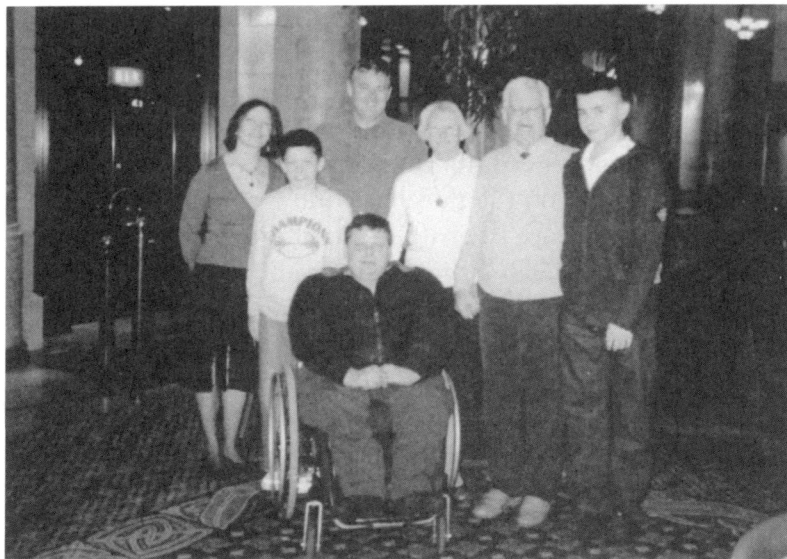

Family – Adrian, Edwina, Trefor, Jill, Huw, Joe and Olly, March 2006

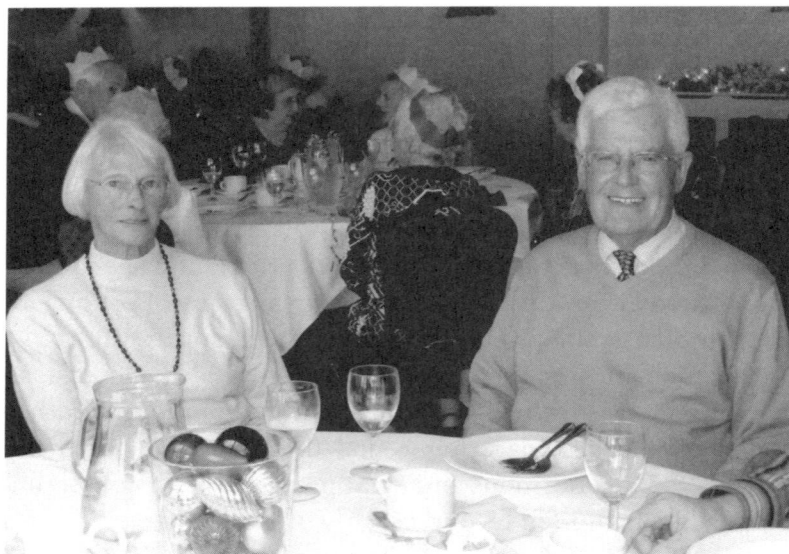

Edwina and I celebrating Christmas with Meeting Point at Thornhill Church

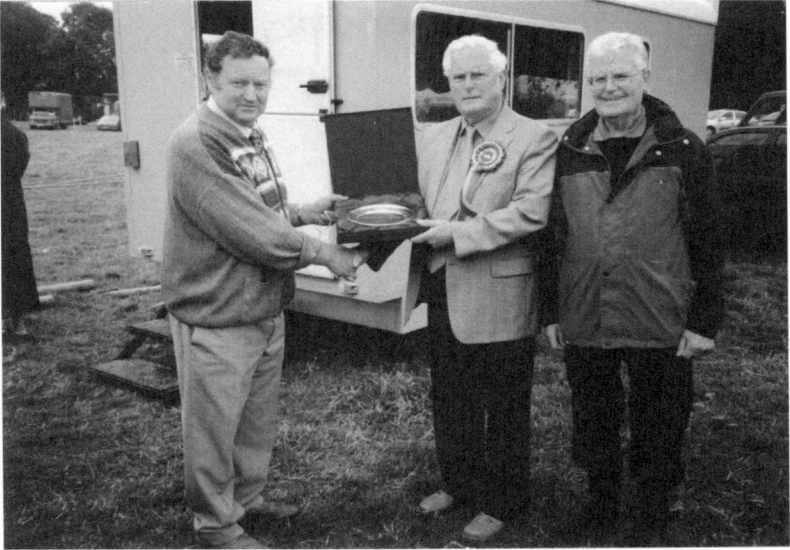

With my brother Trefor who was president of Cilycwm Show in 2004

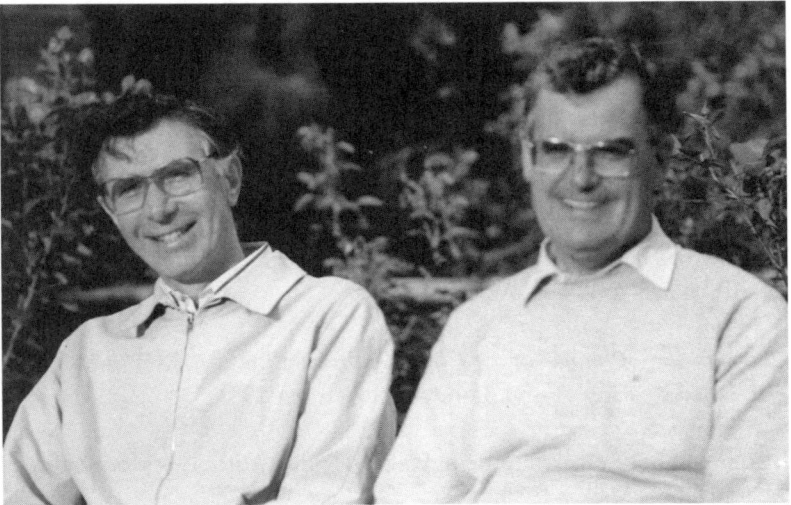

The late Hefin Elias and I, fellow elders and Ardwynians

Appendix

List of other publications, papers etc. by the author

'Transport Management – General Considerations', Association of Chief Ambulance Officers national conference, Harrogate, August 1982.

'Aspects of the 1982 Reorganisation', Association of Welsh Health Authorities annual conference, Llanberis, May 1982.

'Planning and Administrating a Service to achieve Value for Money', conference at Welsh National School of Medicine, Cardiff, April 1982. (Proceedings of the conference *Achieving value for money in medical care* published July 1982.)

'Doctors and Administrators – A New Relationship', symposium for clinicians arranged by Welsh National School of Medicine, October 1981.

'Review of Health Services in Wales', visit by Irish chief executives of health boards to Wales, June 1981.

Closures and Change of Use of Health Facilities. A M Evans et al. Published by King's Fund, London, November 1981.

'Patients First'. Association of Welsh Health Authorities conference, Abergavenny, March 1980.

'The Work of an Area Administrator', King's Fund College, July 1979.

'Administrative Services', management course for clinicians, University College, Cardiff, December 1978.

'Three Years Later – Coming to Terms with Reality', *The Hospital and Health Service Review* (Vol. 73 No. 3), March 1977.

'The Introduction of Medical Developments, Choice of Priorities for the Community Served and Change in the Configuration of Services', international seminar for senior administrators, King's Fund, London. May 1977.

The Role of Psychologists in the Health Service, DHSS, May 1977. Member of the sub-committee set up by the Standing Mental Health Advisory Committee.

'Christianity in Management and Teamwork', national conference at Westminster Central Hall, London, June 1976.

'The Priorities of Health Care', west of England Study Conference, Bristol, November 1975.

'Provision of Health Care Services – Some Aspects of Management', international seminar for senior administrators, King's Fund, London, June 1975.

'NHS – How it Works', advisor on article in *WHICH* magazine, April 1975.

'Problems and Opportunities', *The Hospital and Health Service Review* (Vol. 70 No. 4), April 1975.

Why work as a Manager in the NHS. Film produced by DHSS NHS Training Aids Unit, February 1975.

'Management Organisation – Sector Arrangements', conference of single district teaching areas at Manchester Business School, January 1975.

'Integration of the Health Service', Hotel Catering and Institutional Management Association national conference, Manchester, July 1973.

'NHS Reorganisation and its Implications', Association for Spina Bifida and Hydrocephalus national council, London, June 1973.

'Reorientation towards integration of the Health Service', *The Hospital and Health Service Review* (Vol. 68 No. 100), October 1972.

Report of Working Party on Industrial Relations, member of working party set up by Welsh Hospital Board, May 1972.

'Introducing Changes', Industrial Society (Public Services Group) course, London, September 1971.

'Consultative Document on NHS Reorganisation – Managerial Implications'. South West Metropolitan regional conference, Chertsey, June 1971.

'Management of the Hospital and Group', International Hospital Federation course for overseas administrators, London, March 1971.

'Strategic Planning for Health Services'. University of Manchester Senior Hospital Management course, November 1970.

'The Role of the Chaplain in the Hospital Service', South-west Wales conference, Carmarthen, September 1970.

'The Role of the Voluntary Worker – A Problem Area', third international conference on alcoholism and addiction, Cardiff, September 1970.

'Changing role of the District and General Hospital', British Red Cross regional conference, Usk, September 1970.

'An Administrator's View of Hospital Communications', Student Nurses' Association national conference, Royal College of Nurses, Manchester University, July 1970.

'Reorganisation of the Health Services in Wales – Looking at the Green Paper', national conference, Cardiff, April 1970.

'Developing the Individual in an Organisation', working party on training and administration, Welsh Association for Social Work Development, Cardiff, February 1970.

'Management and Communication' and 'Change in the NHS', seminars for Welsh Hospital Board and HMC members, 1969/70.

'Learning to Think', member of Advanced Management Programmes international course (Harvard Business School) at Swansea University, July/August 1969.

'The Context of Decision Making – Staff Involvement', intensive course for management in the public service, University of Wales Institute of Science and Technology, Cardiff, May 1969.

'Utilising Hospital Resources – The Managerial Mechanism', conference on management in medicine, Royal College of Physicians, London, September 1968.

'Internal Communications in Hospitals', research project sponsored by the King's Fund, Ministry of Health and Guy's Hospital Medical School, to help solve problems of communications and internal management. West Middlesex Hospital report by N F Coghill, A M Evans et al., March 1968.

'Personnel Departments in Public Services', Knight News, October 1967.

'Management of Personnel in the Hospital Service', symposium at King's Fund Centre, London, September 1967.

The Shape of Hospital Management in 1980?, member of the joint working party set up by the King's Fund and the Institute of Hospital Administrators, King's Fund, June 1967.

'The Organisation and Management of Patient Services', Association of Medical Records Officers national conference, Llandudno, May 1967.

'Personnel Policies at Hospital Level', Ministry of Health, London, April 1966.

'The Hospital Secretary', course for overseas administrators, King's Fund Centre, March 1966.

'The Organisation of Outpatient Departments and the Ambulance Service', Association of Ambulance Officers national conference, Eastbourne, October 1965.

'Management Problems from a Unit Administrator's Viewpoint', Institute of Hospital Administrators (Sheffield Region) annual conference, Nottingham University, September 1965.

'Management of Hospital and Health Services – an evaluation and a concept', *The Hospital* (Vol. 61 No. 3), March 1965.

'Work Study in a Medical Records Department', Association of Medical Records Officers conference, Swansea, June 1964.

Survey of Male Portering Staff in the Hospital Service (based on interviews of head porters and 100 porters at seven hospitals in the south Wales area) – in collaboration with W D Morgan, AHA, Welsh Staff Advisory Committee, April 1964.

'Research on Hospital Outpatient and Casualty Attendance' in collaboration with John Wakeford, BA, University College, Cardiff in *The Hospital* (Vol. 60 No. 4), April 1964.

'Work Study in the NHS', Institute of Hospital Administrators (Welsh Region) annual conference, Porthcawl, September 1962.

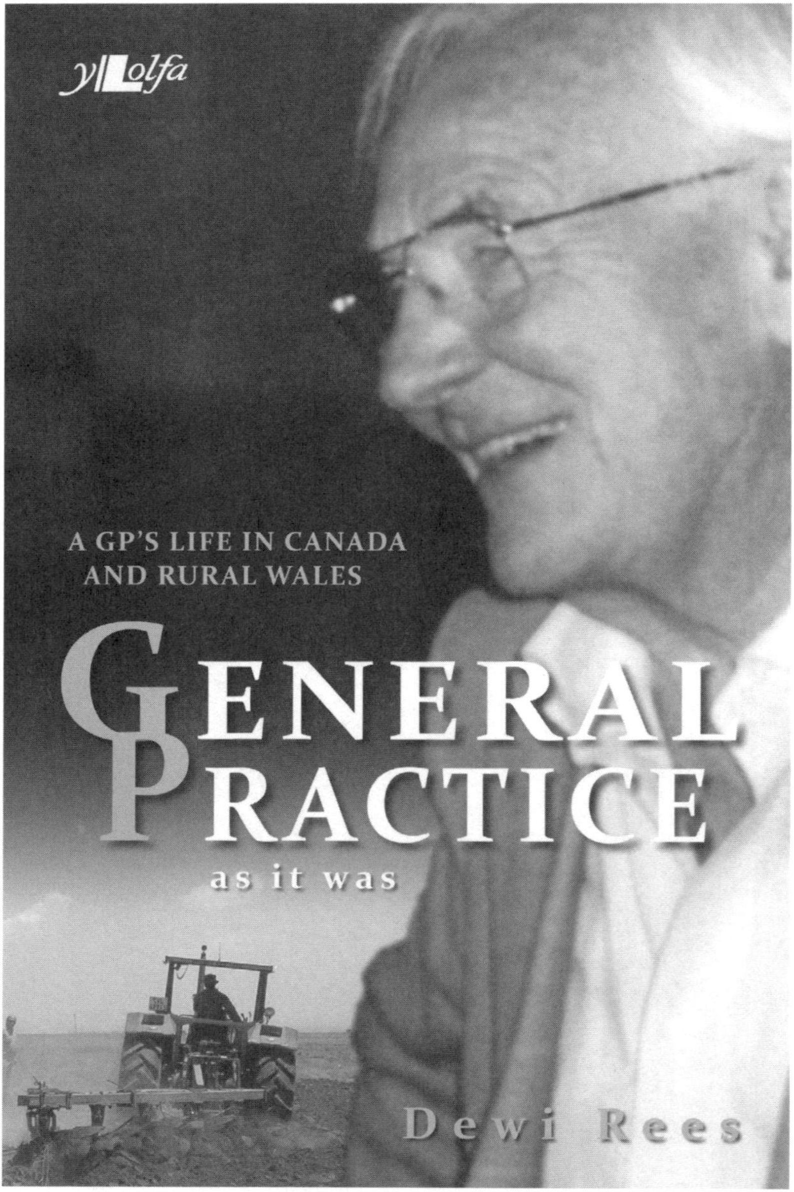
y Lolfa
A GP'S LIFE IN CANADA
AND RURAL WALES
GENERAL
PRACTICE
as it was
Dewi Rees

£9.95

Joshua Gerwyn Elias

A Doctor's Tale

yLolfa

£7.95

A Life's Journey is just one of a whole range of publications from Y Lolfa. For a full list of books currently in print, send now for your free copy of our new full-colour catalogue. Or simply surf into our website

www.ylolfa.com

for secure on-line ordering.

yLolfa

TALYBONT CEREDIGION CYMRU SY24 5HE
e-mail ylolfa@ylolfa.com
website www.ylolfa.com
phone (01970) 832 304
fax 832 782